There's an entire world of reliable research-based scientific information about preventing illness and treating disease with safe natural substances—vitamins, minerals, botanicals, and other things—that's being deliberately hidden from you! If you prefer patent medicines ("pharmaceuticals"), you are also being deliberately prevented from accessing them at the very best prices. No, I'm not kidding or exaggerating at all. If all of this information were made freely available, and barriers to access were eliminated, the cost of healthcare would drop dramatically within just a few years, and both as individuals and a nation, we'd be much healthier with much less expense.

Bill Faloon's *Pharmocracy* details exactly why this enormous amount of information is being withheld, and describes precisely how it is being done, despite our Constitutional guarantee of freedom of speech and freedom of the press. He writes about the "barriers to access" to less expensive patent medicines ("pharmaceuticals"). Please read this book if you want to know why—despite miracle surgeries and diagnostic techniques—American healthcare is much more costly and less effective than it could be if we truly had freedom of choice, freedom of information and freedom of access here in these United States of America.

Pharmocracy doesn't just detail these problems, it gives us the solutions. If you want access to this vast amount of reliable information and less expensive treatments that will help you and your family stay as healthy as you can as long as you can, please read this book and take action! Together we can get it done.

—JONATHAN V. WRIGHT, MD

Pharmocracy

Pharmocracy

*How Corrupt Deals and Misguided Medical
Regulations Are Bankrupting America—
and What to Do About It*

William Faloon
Co-founder of the
Life Extension Foundation®

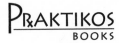

PRAKTIKOS
BOOKS

IMPORTANT NOTICE

This book contains financial data spanning several decades that describes the impending insolvency of Medicare and other government-related health programs. Due to various accounting gimmicks employed by Congress and federal agencies, there are considerable fluctuations from year to year, such as whether Medicare's true unfunded liability is $24.6 or $37 trillion. Likewise, the prices of prescription drugs rapidly change, so drug costs stated in this book may be higher or lower at any given time in the future. The author has striven to present an accurate picture of this financial situation based on available information, but inconsistencies in reporting and varying interpretations have created a potentially large margin of error.

DISCLAIMER

Ideas and information in this book are based upon the experience and training of the author and the scientific information currently available. The suggestions in this book are definitely not meant to be a substitute for careful medical evaluation and treatment by a qualified, licensed health professional. The author and publisher do not recommend changing or adding medication or supplements without consulting your personal physician. They specifically disclaim any liability arising directly or indirectly from the use of this book.

Praktikos Books
P.O. Box 118
Mount Jackson, VA 22842
888.542.9467   info@praktikosbooks.com

Praktikos Books are produced in alliance with Axios Press.

Library of Congress Cataloging-in-Publication Data

Faloon, William.
    Pharmocracy : how corrupt deals and misguided medical regulations are bankrupting America—and what to do about it / William Faloon.
    p. cm.
    Includes bibliographical references and index.
    ISBN 978-1-60766-011-8 (hardcover)
    1. Medical care—United States. 2. Drugs—Costs. 3. Budget deficits—United States. 4. United States. Food and Drug Administration. 5. Medical policy—United States. I. Title.
RA410.53.F35 2011
338.4'76151–dc23

2011024233

Contents

Preface

EALTHCARE IS BANKRUPTING the United States. Medical costs have escalated to a level that individuals, businesses, and debt-laden governments can no longer afford to pay for it.

There is a real-world solution.

Congress can create new legislation that will allow free-market forces to drive down sick care costs, better enable disease prevention, and rapidly perfect curative therapies.

This book provides factual documentation on just how broken the US healthcare system is today. It is over 300 pages long because there are at least that many reasons why healthcare costs far more than it should.

Until now, no one has identified and amalgamated the plethora of illogical regulations that directly cause healthcare to be so overpriced.

While this book attacks FDA corruption and ineptitude, Congress is the body of government that provides the FDA with enabling laws that ultimately result in needless suffering and death—while the nation descends into financial ruination.

Implementing free-market approaches can spare Medicare and Medicaid from insolvency, while significantly improving the health and productivity of the American public.

Pharmocracy provides an irrefutable and rational basis to remove the suffocating compulsory aspect of healthcare regulation and allow free-market forces to compete against government-sanctioned medicine.

This book documents how the free market can provide superior healthcare at far lower prices while better protecting consumers.

I fear that disregard of the obvious problems revealed in this book will condemn the United States to a downward economic spiral with little improvement in human longevity.

Introduction

AFIERCE DEBATE IS RAGING as to *who* will pay for this nation's skyrocketing "sick-care" costs.

Private companies have scaled back sharply on the healthcare coverage they used to provide.[1,2] Employees now pay an increasing percentage of their medical insurance premiums, along with higher deductibles, co-pays, and no-pays (i.e., exclusions). Many businesses provide their employees with *no* health coverage.

Based on the median income in the United States, the typical family cannot come close to paying the staggering cost of healthcare themselves.

It seems rather odd, but since neither the private business sector nor individuals can afford today's sick-care costs, the burden is increasingly being borne by the sector *least* able to pay, i.e., heavily indebted local, state, and federal governments.

Even those covered by government insurance (such as retired veterans, municipal employees, and Medicare recipients) are facing higher medical insurance premiums.

The federal government is already saddled with a huge *unfunded* Medicare liability. No one has figured out where the money will come from to cover these future healthcare costs.

To put Medicare alone into context, the unfunded liability is now $24.6 trillion.[3] Yet total federal tax revenue taken in annually (which includes Medicare premiums) is only around $2 trillion.[4, 5] As our president stated in 2010, we are approaching a point where government will have to spend more money on Medicare than on every other federal program combined![6, 7]

This does not count the escalating costs of Medicaid (sick-care coverage for the poor) that are shared by federal and state governments. Medicaid is funded with current tax revenue and newly issued debt, but its spiraling growth has created a new multi-trillion dollar unfunded liability, and no one knows where the money will come from to pay it.[8]

Bernard Madoff was sentenced to 150 years in prison because he took investors' money and diverted it to other purposes. The federal government forced Americans to pay Medicare premiums their entire lives. Instead of those premiums being placed in a reserve fund for future use, they were squandered on whatever was most politically expedient at the time, which included overpaying—with tax dollars—those with the right connections.

While Madoff will spend the rest of his life incarcerated, no one talks about bringing civil or criminal charges against those responsible for the largest Ponzi scheme in the history of the human race: Medicare, with its $24.6 trillion of unfunded liabilities.

Like the federal government, many local and state governments have also operated a Ponzi scheme of unfunded pension and healthcare liabilities they cannot pay. Since the federal government is mathematically insolvent, it seems ludicrous to assume that exorbitant sick-care costs can be resolved by any level of government.

While politicians aimlessly point fingers over who should pay America's medical bills, please remember that there is a real-world solution. Healthcare in the United States is so tightly regulated that it in many ways resembles the inefficiencies of Maoist China, where the economy suffocated for decades from erratic and illogical governmental decrees. As China lifted its regulatory stranglehold, prosperity flourished. It's time for US leaders to follow China's example and stop over-regulating medicine!

EVEN THE AUTHOR WAS SHOCKED

The non-profit Life Extension Foundation® has sounded the alarm bells since the early 1980s about the healthcare cost crisis we now face. We said that unless the shackles of regulation are removed, this nation would face inevitable economic insolvency, with little in the way of cures being found for age-related diseases.

I have written dozens of articles and made hundreds of media appearances attacking today's broken healthcare system. I was not aware until recently, however, of how much my own health insurance premiums had gone up, since I was covered under a group plan.

For my wife, two children, and me, the Life Extension® organization I co-founded is paying a staggering $17,000 every year! Since our group plan insures over 300 people, we obtain a considerable discount off the individual rate—yet the premiums, deductibles, co-pays, and no-pays are worse than ever.

I'd like to think the Life Extension Foundation® is the most efficiently run organization in the world, as we have gone to great strides to ensure our perpetual existence. Life Extension® can at the moment afford these outrageous health insurance premiums for our dedicated employees. But I know many businesses and individuals cannot, and certainly the government cannot, since it is unable to afford what it is already on the hook for.

WE HAVE BEEN DECEIVED BY BIG PHARMA

Look back over the past 30 years and ask: How many cures for the diseases of aging have been found? One can argue the number is near zero!

Americans have paid outlandish prices for prescription drugs believing that pharmaceutical profits would fund research leading to medical breakthroughs. The problem is that real-world discoveries have not manifested themselves. One can point to some treatments that prolong patient survival, but these are offset by lethal side effects inflicted by fraudulently approved therapies.[9-11] The fact is that few real cures have occurred, despite Americans spending more healthcare dollars than anyone else.

Examples of cures are antibiotics and vaccines that eradicated diseases. These were developed long before today's regulatory stranglehold ended these kinds of breakthrough innovations.

Unregulated medicine has made considerable strides, but the majority of the population does not know about these approaches, and vested financial interests have spent billions to ensure that the media, politicians, and bureaucrats continue suppressing them.

Americans have been deceived by those who associate regulations with beneficial outcomes. As it relates to medical progress, the opposite has occurred.[12]

Few understand that the underlying purpose of any given regulation is to provide a government-protected advantage to the group favoring that regulation. It's not about how a regulation will protect the public, but instead a matter of "how can it financially benefit a special interest."[13]

An oft-cited example is a petition the drug maker Wyeth filed with the FDA asking that a natural human form of estrogen called estriol be banned.[14] The female hormone drugs Wyeth is selling (Premarin® and PremPro®) had been shown to inflict all kinds of lethal side effects.[15-24] Instead of spending money on research to come up with safer forms of estrogen (such as combining natural estrogens with indole-3-carbinol),[25-31] it was much cheaper to persuade political hacks at the FDA to outlaw the competition (i.e., bioidentical estriol hormone compounds).[32]

Pharmaceutical companies have spent enormous amounts of money persuading the FDA to reclassify nutrients like pyridoxamine into prescription drugs so they can monopolize them for their own economic benefit.[33] If it were not for aggressive letter-writing campaigns by consumers to Congress, *all* dietary supplements would be expensive prescription drugs by now.

FDA—FAILURE, DECEPTION, ABUSE

In 2010, we released a 498-page book called *FDA: Failure, Deception, Abuse*, which exposed how over-regulation has destroyed citizens' health and this nation's finances. This book, *Pharmocracy*, provides startling updates to a medical crisis that is exploding out of control.

The magnitude of the artificially inflated costs are beyond obscene. For example, an increasingly popular prescription drug in the United States is a testosterone ointment called AndroGel®. Last time we checked, pharmacy chains sell a one-month supply for $348. Many men who try it will continue to use it each month for the rest of their lives.

The cost of the active ingredient in AndroGel® is around $4.00. It costs a few more dollars to put it into ointment form under good manufacturing practices. So for less than $15.00 retail, consumers could purchase this same amount of testosterone—if it were not for FDA over-regulation.

Even though transdermal testosterone delivery technology has been around for decades, and the patent for bioidentical testosterone expired forever ago, the FDA only
allows a chosen few pharmaceutical companies to sell it.
When a compounding pharmacy tries to develop more efficient ways of making testosterone creams, FDA inspectors
use existing regulations to stop them. These regulations
mandate that individually compounded drugs be made
from scratch. If a pharmacy tries to produce larger quantities in bulk, it is no longer classified as "compounded"
according to FDA regulations and therefore illegal.[34]

In this Orwellian tragedy, the annual cost of regulated
AndroGel® comes to $4,176, whereas the same amount of
topical testosterone in an unregulated environment would
drop to only $180 a year.

Regulated testosterone thus costs 23 times more than
free-market testosterone. And look who pays for it! If
you have health insurance, you will likely have to fork
over $25 to $50 co-pay each month, while your insurance company is fleeced for the balance. If you are a low
income individual and don't have insurance, there are
government programs (like Medicaid) that will pay the
full retail price of AndroGel®. If you are not indigent and
have no insurance, then you are stuck with the entire tab.
Whether you are a taxpayer, co-payer, or out-of-pocket
payer, your finances are being eaten away by these absurd
regulations. Is it any wonder why medical insurance premiums are increasing so sharply?

Now imagine someone in Congress introducing a bill
repealing this kind of FDA-protected monopoly. The
pharmaceutical industry would spend whatever amount
of money it would take to keep this law from being
enacted, and would heavily finance whoever ran against

this member of Congress in the next election. In other words, it would be political suicide to attempt to allow unregulated drugs to be sold, even though deregulation would go a long way to solving today's healthcare cost crisis. That's why consumers have to band together to demand Congress ignore pharmaceutical lobbyists and introduce emergency legislation that repeals the absurd over-regulation of medicine that exists today.

The title of this book is *Pharmocracy*, but I contemplated the original title as *Regulation Breeds Corruption*. The reason I considered that title is that egregious pharmaceutical company profits are protected by regulations, and these vested interests will go to any corrupt length to ensure these regulations are perpetuated, no matter how inane they are.[35,36]

The word "corruption" is often interpreted as meaning something illegal. The word corruption, however, can be defined as immoral behavior, an example of which is the exploitation of a position of power for personal gain. When it comes to campaign contributions, lobbying, and offering congressional staff generous employment after they retire, these are not overtly illegal acts.[37] They routinely happen, which means this kind of devastating corruption has been institutionalized.

HOW REGULATED COSTS ADD UP

Institutionalized corruption artificially inflates the cost of virtually every healthcare service.

Going back to the AndroGel® example, we estimate that more than 80 million American men could benefit by restoring their testosterone levels to youthful ranges.[38] If these men are forced to use only FDA-approved testosterone drugs, the excess cost to the United States will be $319 billion each year for this one drug.

As recently as a few years ago, when the entire federal deficit reached $300 billion, the public and some politicians complained. Yet the overpayment Americans are stuck with for this one class of drug (AndroGel® and others) because of FDA over-regulation may exceed previous federal deficits unless the law is amended.

When one considers there are thousands of medical-related products and services that are artificially inflated by senseless regulations, it becomes clear that radical change is required to avoid an economic meltdown.

EVEN COMPOUNDED TESTOSTERONE COSTS TOO MUCH

As stated earlier, FDA regulations prohibit compounding pharmacies from making production-scale batches of popular drugs. Each compounded drug must be individually formulated by a licensed pharmacist. The result is the labor involved in making a compounded drug costs more than the active ingredient itself.

But there are additional regulations that result in even greater costs. Consumers require a prescription to buy compounded testosterone, just like they do FDA-approved testosterone. While competent physician supervision can enhance the safety and efficacy of a testosterone replacement program, the frank reality is that the majority of prescriptions for drugs like AndroGel® are prescribed by physicians who know very little about how to optimally manage hormone replacement in men. For instance, estrogen levels are seldom monitored in order to protect against estrogen overload, which can occur when too much testosterone converts (aromatizes) into estrogen in an aging man's body.[39,40]

An advantage of compounded testosterone is that a physician who knows how to write a prescription for it will often have received training on follow-up monitoring. Compounded testosterone cream can be obtained for less than $30 a month, compared to the $348/month price for AndroGel®. Either form can contain the same amount of bioidentical testosterone.

Compounded testosterone cream is 91% less expensive than FDA-protected drugs, yet compounded testosterone is still twice as expensive as it needs to be because of governmental over-regulation.

In dealing with runaway healthcare costs, a solution is to make drugs like testosterone available to men over age 40 without the necessity of a doctor's visit. There have been companies that have physicians review blood tests over the phone and prescribe testosterone, but the FDA and state licensing boards have shut many of them down.[41]

Corrupt regulations ensure that efficiencies that would slash healthcare costs (at the expense of extortionist pharmaceutical profits) never see the light of day.

SIMPLE SOLUTION TO AVERT ECONOMIC RUINATION

The Life Extension Foundation® initiated a petition drive back in the 1980s to allow individual Americans to "opt out" of the FDA's regulatory umbrella. Our rationale was that this would provide consumers with more advanced treatments at lower prices.

Hundreds of enlightened Life Extension Foundation® members petitioned the FDA demanding liberation from its regulatory stranglehold. The public, Congress, and the media were apathetic at that time.

The FDA was far from lethargic. They responded to our petition in a way that resembled an angry hornet's nest when disturbed (or how some dictators respond to street protestors). The notion that we dared challenge the FDA's absolute authority resulted in years of legal battles where the FDA did everything in its power to try to destroy the Life Extension Foundation® (and put me in jail).[42]

Fast-forward to today. The political climate has changed. The healthcare cost crisis we long ago predicted has evolved into a harsh reality no one can ignore. It is mathematically impossible to solve it by forcing one group to pay regulated medicine's corrupt inflated costs. The only salvation is the free-market reforms that the Life Extension Foundation® long ago drafted.

Our proposal is quite simple. Change the laws to allow good manufacturing practice (GMP)-certified manufacturing facilities to produce generic prescription drugs that do not undergo the excessive regulatory hurdles that force consumers to pay egregiously inflated prices.

To alert consumers when they are getting a generic that is not as heavily regulated as it is currently, the law would mandate that the label of these less-regulated generic drugs clearly state:

> This is not an FDA-approved manufactured generic drug and may be ineffective and potentially dangerous. This drug is not manufactured under the same standards required for an FDA-approved generic drug. Purchase this drug at your own risk.

By allowing the sale of these less costly generics, consumers will have a choice as to which companies they choose to trust.

Equally important among our proposals is one that allows consumers to be told about the off-label benefits of prescription drugs. An example is the extensive body of evidence that metformin may help prevent—not simply treat—type 2 diabetes,[43,44] and that metformin may also prevent and help treat certain cancers.[45-56]

A concern critics raise about this free-market solution is safety. Who will protect consumers from poorly made generic drugs, they ask?

First of all, the manufacturers of these drugs would be subject to the same regulation as GMP-certified dietary supplement makers. FDA inspectors will visit facilities, take sample products, and assay them to ensure the potency of active ingredients, dissolution, etc. Laboratories that fail to make products which meet the label's claims would face civil and criminal penalties from the government.

Secondly, there is no incentive not to provide the full potency of active ingredients in these less-regulated generic drugs. The price of the active ingredient makes up such a small percentage of the overall cost that a manufacturer would be idiotic to scrimp on potency.[57]

Companies that foolishly make inferior generics will be viciously exposed by the media, along with the FDA, consumer protection groups, and even prescribing physicians who will be suspicious if a drug is not working as it is supposed to.

Companies producing inferior products will be quickly driven from the marketplace as consumers who choose to purchase these lower-cost generics will seek out laboratories that have reputations for making flawless products.

Substandard companies would not only be castigated in the public's eye, but face civil litigation from customers who bought the defective generics. When one considers that GMP-certified manufacturing plants can cost hundreds of millions of dollars to set up, a company would guarantee itself future insolvency if it failed to produce generic drugs that met minimum standards.

PHARMACEUTICAL COMPANY PROPAGANDA

No matter how many facts show that free-market generic drugs will be safe, there are alarmists who believe that even if one person might suffer a serious adverse event because of a lower-cost generic drug, the law should not be amended to allow the sale of these less-regulated products.

What few understand is that enabling lower-cost drugs to be sold might reduce the number of poorly made drugs. The reason is that prescription drug counterfeiting is a major issue today.[58] Drugs are counterfeited because they are so expensive. Yet in the free-market environment we espouse, a month's supply of a popular cholesterol-lowering drug like simvastatin would sell for less than $3.00. It is difficult to imagine anyone profiting by counterfeiting it. So amending the law to enable these super-low-cost drugs to be sold might reduce the counterfeiting that exists right now.

Another reason these less-regulated generics will do far more good than harm is that people who need them to live will be able to afford them. The media has reported on heart-wrenching stories of destitute people who are unable to pay for their prescription drugs. They either do without, or take a less-than-optimal dose. The availability of these free-market generics will enable virtually anyone to be able to afford their medications out of pocket.

AS THIS BOOK WAS BEING FINALIZED . . .

Each chapter in *Pharmocracy* will enlighten you to a new atrocity committed against our health and wealth by today's corrupt regulatory environment.

As this book was being finalized, news broke that the FDA had granted an exclusive monopoly to a company to sell a non-patented progesterone drug that prevents premature births.[59]

Healthy women naturally secrete huge amounts of progesterone during pregnancy, which helps maintain their uterine lining. To protect against premature births and miscarriages in women who don't secrete enough progesterone, doctors have for decades prescribed progesterone medications that were made by state-licensed compounding pharmacies. The cost per injection was around $20.

By granting orphan drug status to one company (KV Pharmaceutical), FDA rules banned all other forms of progesterone for this indication. The immediate impact was that the cost per injection of this progesterone drug was set to skyrocket to $1,500—or as much as $30,000 for a full-term pregnancy.[60]

An uprising over this price gouging forced FDA to back down and state it "does not intend to take enforcement action against pharmacies that compound hydroxyprogesterone caproate."[61]

What the FDA is saying is that while it has the discretion to arrest compounding pharmacists for making this drug, it does not "intend to" do so. After FDA made this announcement, KV Pharmaceutical reduced the price to $690 per injection[62]—which is still more than 34 times its previous free-market price.

It is unclear how private insurance and Medicaid will determine whether to pay $690 per injection for the version the FDA rules state is the only one that can be legally sold, or continue paying for the much lower-cost compounded version.

Women who are denied access to this drug because of this regulatory quagmire face increased risks they will deliver pre-term babies. In these cases, the costs for intensive neonatal care can run into the hundreds of thousands of dollars per prematurely born baby, a price often borne by Medicaid or private insurance.

No country on earth can afford this kind of institutionalized corruption in which the chosen few pharmaceutical companies favored by the FDA reap extortionist profits as the nation collapses into a financial abyss.

This rare instance in which public backlash forced the FDA to back away from protecting a drug company's obscene profit reveals that citizens have the power to save this country from financial Armageddon.

FIGHT BACK AGAINST THIS INSTITUTIONAL CORRUPTION

The United States of America faces a healthcare cost crisis that will render Medicare, Medicaid, and many private insurance plans insolvent. The shocking details about this country's inability to fund medical costs are no longer confined to the pages of *Life Extension Magazine*®. You are reading about them virtually every day in the mainstream media.[63, 64]

When terrorists attacked the United States in 2001, there were patriotic Americans who enlisted in the armed services. Many lost their limbs, their vision, and their lives.

No one has to engage in physical combat to save this country from the institutionalized inefficiencies and corruption that plague today's disease care system. All you have to do is type www.lef.org/lac into your computer's web browser, and you can easily send a copy of these introductory chapters and a special letter to your representative and two senators.

It is that simple to take affirmative action to help save our country from the insolvency so many other countries chronically suffer with.

I sincerely hope that after reading this book, not one reader will fail to email his or her congressional representative and senators at www.lef.org/lac.

We must unite and demand that Congress tear down the barriers of medical over-regulation that are destroying this nation's financial future.

UPDATE

In 2009, Medicare's unfunded liability was pegged at $37 trillion.[65] What that means is that for the government to meet its future obligations, it should have had $37 trillion in a trust fund earning interest. But politicians constantly manipulate the numbers. The latest report[3] stated that the Medicare unfunded liability was $24.6 trillion. The reason for these wild fluctuations is that in any given year, government officials can create "assumptions" out of thin air, like assuming doctors will take 21% pay cuts. Congress has not enacted these mandatory pay cuts, but bureaucrats sometimes pretend they have so that Medicare's true unfunded liability is understated. Despite these accounting gimmicks, the government's most recent report released in 2011 states that Medicare's hospital fund will go bankrupt in 2024, which is five years sooner than Medicare's trustees estimated the prior year. Be it $24 trillion or $37 trillion, the government does not have the money to pay for its Medicare obligations. Nor does it have the money to cover its unfunded liabilities for Medicaid, veterans, or federal employee health plans—nor the trillions of additional sick-care dollars it is on the hook for.

References

1. Available at: http://www.sciencedaily.com/releases/2009/08/090818182051.htm. Accessed March 24, 2011.
2. Available at: http://www.csmonitor.com/2003/1028/p01s02-usec.html. Accessed March 24, 2011.
3. Medical Trustees 2011 Annual Report. Department of Health and Human Services, Baltimore, MD. May 13, 2011.

4. Available at: http://www.gao.gov/financial/fy2010/10frusg. pdf. Accessed March 24, 2011.

5. Available at: http://www.taxpolicycenter.org/taxfacts/ displayafact.cfm?Docid=407. Accessed March 24, 2011.

6. Available at: http://www.whitehouse.gov/the_press_office/ remarks-by-the-president-to-a-joint-session-of-congress-on-health-care. Accessed March 24, 2011.

7. Available at: http://www.ncpa.org/pub/ba662. Accessed March 24, 2011.

8. Available at: http://www.glgroup.com/News/If-you-think-health-care-and-Medicare-are-problems-consider-long-term-care-and-Medicaid.-30757.html. Accessed March 24, 2011.

9. Available at: http://yourwisdom.yahoo.com/your-health/ avastin-cancer-treatment-drug-actually-raises-risk-death-article-acid.html. Accessed March 24, 2011.

10. Available at: http://www.pcrm.org/newsletter/aug10/diabetes_ drugs.html. Accessed March 24, 2011.

11. Ranpura V, Hapani S, Wu S. Treatment-related mortality with bevacizumab in cancer patients: a meta-analysis. *JAMA.* 2011 Feb 2;305(5):487–94.

12. Available at: http://rutherfordtimesonline.com/2010/03/09/ the-audacity-of-freedom-government-regulation-of-the-pharmaceutical-industry-harms-more-than-helps. Accessed March 24, 2011.

13. Available at: http://www.progressiveradionetwork.com/ health-headlines/2010/7/16/special-report-pharmaceutical-profit-big-government-and-bias.html. Accessed March 24, 2011.

14. Available at: http://www.anh-usa.org/access-to-estriol-2/. Accessed March 24, 2011.

15. Rossouw JE, Anderson GL, Prentice RL, et al. Risks and benefits of estrogen plus progestin in healthy postmenopausal women: principal results From the Women's Health Initiative randomized controlled trial. *JAMA.* 2002 Jul 17;288(3):321–33.

16. Vongpatanasin W, Tuncel M, Wang Z, Arbique D, Mehrad B, Jialal I. Differential effects of oral versus transdermal estrogen replacement therapy on C-reactive protein in postmenopausal women. *J Am Coll Cardiol.* 2003 Apr 16;41(8):1358–63.

17. Chen CL, Weiss NS, Newcomb P, Barlow W, White E. Hormone replacement therapy in relation to breast cancer. *JAMA*. 2002 Feb 13;287(6):734–41.

18. Beral V. Breast cancer and hormone-replacement therapy in the Million Women Study. *Lancet*. 2003 Aug 9;362(9382):419–27.

19. Cushman M, Kuller LH, Prentice R, et al. Estrogen plus progestin and risk of venous thrombosis. *JAMA*. 2004 Oct 6;292(13):1573–80.

20. Anderson GL, Judd HL, Kaunitz AM, et al. Effects of estrogen plus progestin on gynecologic cancers and associated diagnostic procedures: the Women's Health Initiative randomized trial. *JAMA*. 2003 Oct 1;290(13):1739–48.

21. Manson JE, Hsia J, Johnson KC, et al. Estrogen plus progestin and the risk of coronary heart disease. *N Engl J Med*. 2003 Aug 7;349(6):523–34.

22. Shumaker SA, Legault C, Rapp SR, et al. Estrogen plus progestin and the incidence of dementia and mild cognitive impairment in postmenopausal women: the Women's Health Initiative Memory Study: a randomized controlled trial. *JAMA*. 2003 May 28;289(20):2651–62.

23. Maalouf NM, Sato AH, Welch BJ, et al. Postmenopausal hormone use and the risk of nephrolithiasis: results from the Women's Health Initiative hormone therapy trials. *Arch Intern Med*. 2010 Oct 11;170(18):1678–85.

24. Slatore CG, Chien JW, Au DH, Satia JA, White E. Lung cancer and hormone replacement therapy: association in the vitamins and lifestyle study. *J Clin Oncol*. 2010 Mar 20;28(9):1540–6.

25. Weng JR, Tsai CH, Kulp SK, Chen CS. Indole-3-carbinol as a chemopreventive and anti-cancer agent. *Cancer Lett*. 2008 Apr 18;262(2):153–63.

26. Auborn KJ, Fan S, Rosen EM, et al. Indole-3-carbinol is a negative regulator of estrogen. *J Nutr*. 2003 Jul;133(7 Suppl):2470S–2475S.

27. Ashok BT, Chen YG, Liu X, et al. Multiple molecular targets of indole-3-carbinol, a chemopreventive anti-estrogen in breast cancer. *Eur J Cancer Prev*. 2002 Aug;11 Suppl 2S86-S93.

28. Yuan F, Chen DZ, Liu K, et al. Anti-estrogenic activities of indole-3-carbinol in cervical cells: implication for prevention of cervical cancer. *Anticancer Res.* 1999 May;19(3A):1673–80.

29. Bell MC, Crowley-Nowick P, Bradlow HL, et al. Placebo-controlled trial of indole-3-carbinol in the treatment of CIN. *Gynecol Oncol.* 2000 Aug;78(2):123–9.

30. Nakamura Y, Yogosawa S, Izutani Y, Watanabe H, Otsuji E, Sakai T. A combination of indol-3-carbinol and genistein synergistically induces apoptosis in human colon cancer HT-29 cells by inhibiting Akt phosphorylation and progression of autophagy. *Mol Cancer.* 2009 Nov 12; 8:100.

31. Fowke JH, Longcope C, Hebert JR. Brassica vegetable consumption shifts estrogen metabolism in healthy postmenopausal women. *Cancer Epidemiol Biomarkers Prev.* 2000 Aug;9(8):773–9.

32. Available at: http://www.anh-usa.org/bioidentical-estriol-still-under-threat/. Accessed March 25, 2011.

33. Faloon W. FDA seeks to ban pyridoxamine. *Life Extension Magazine®.* 2009 Jul;15(7):7–12.

34. Available at: http://www.fda.gov/NewsEvents/Newsroom/PressAnnouncements/2008/ucm116832.htm. Accessed March 25, 2011.

35. Available at: http://articles.mercola.com/sites/articles/archive/2011/03/22/betrayal-of-consumers-by-us-supreme-court-gives-total-liability-shield-to-big-pharma.aspx. Accessed March 25, 2011.

36. Available at: http://www.pharmalot.com/2007/04/60_minutes_beats_up_big_pharma/. Accessed March 25, 2011.

37. Available at: http://www.publicintegrity.org/hiredguns/. Accessed March 25, 2011.

38. Faloon W. Startling low testosterone blood levels in male Life Extension® members. *Life Extension Magazine®.* 2010 Jun;16(6):7–14.

39. Vermeulen A, Kaufman JM, Goemaere S, van Pottelberg I. Estradiol in elderly men. *Aging Male.* 2002 Jun;5(2):98–102.

40. Cohen PG. Aromatase, adiposity, aging and disease. The hypogonadal-metabolic-atherogenic-disease and aging connection. *Med Hypotheses.* 2001 Jun;56(6):702–8.

41. Available at: http://www.acpinternist.org/archives/1999/11/ epharm.htm. Accessed March 25, 2011.

42. Available at: http://www.benbest.com/polecon/fdalef.html. Accessed March 25, 2011.

43. Zinman B, Harris SB, Neuman J, et al. Low-dose combination therapy with rosiglitazone and metformin to prevent type 2 diabetes mellitus (CANOE trial): a double-blind randomised controlled study. *Lancet.* 2010 Jul 10;376(9735):103–11.

44. Charles MA, Eschwege E. Prevention of type 2 diabetes: Role of metformin. *Drugs.* 1999;58 Suppl.1:71–3.

45. Libby G, Donnelly LA, Donnan PT, Alessi DR, Morris AD, Evans JM. New users of metformin are at low risk of incident cancer: a cohort study among people with type 2 diabetes. *Diabetes Care.* 2009 Sep;32(9):1620–5.

46. Rattan R, Giri S, Hartmann L, Shridhar V. Metformin attenuates ovarian cancer cell growth in an AMP-kinase dispensable manner. *J Cell Mol Med.* 2011 Jan;15(1):166–78.

47. Liu B, Fan Z, Edgerton SM, et al. Metformin induces unique biological and molecular responses in triple negative breast cancer cells. *Cell Cycle.* 2009 Jul 1;8(13):2031–40.

48. Anisimov VN, Egormin PA, Piskunova TS, et al. Metformin extends life span of HER-2/neu transgenic mice and in combination with melatonin inhibits growth of transplantable tumors in vivo. *Cell Cycle.* 2010 Jan 1;9(1):188–97.

49. Alimova IN, Liu B, Fan Z, et al. Metformin inhibits breast cancer cell growth, colony formation and induces cell cycle arrest in vitro. *Cell Cycle.* 2009 Mar 15;8(6):909–15.

50. Bodmer M, Meier C, Krahenbuhl S, Jick SS, Meier CR. Long-term metformin use is associated with decreased risk of breast cancer. *Diabetes Care.* 2010 Jun;33(6):1304–8.

51. Yurekli BS, Karaca B, Cetinkalp S, Uslu R. Is it the time for metformin to take place in adjuvant treatment of Her-2 positive breast cancer? Teaching new tricks to old dogs. *Med Hypotheses.* 2009 Oct;73(4):606–7.

52. Stanosz S. An attempt at conservative treatment in selected cases of type I endometrial carcinoma (stage I a/G1) in young women. *Eur J Gynaecol Oncol.* 2009;30(4):365–9.

53. Ben Sahra I, Laurent K, Giuliano S, et al. Targeting cancer cell metabolism: the combination of metformin and 2-deoxyglucose

induces p53-dependent apoptosis in prostate cancer cells. *Cancer Res.* 2010 Mar 15;70(6):2465-75.

54. Wang LW, Li ZS, Zou DW, Jin ZD, Gao J, Xu GM. Metformin induces apoptosis of pancreatic cancer cells. *World J Gastroenterol.* 2008 Dec 21;14(47):7192-8.

55. Algire C, Amrein L, Zakikhani M, Panasci L, Pollak M. Metformin blocks the stimulative effect of a high-energy diet on colon carcinoma growth in vivo and is associated with reduced expression of fatty acid synthase. *Endocr Relat Cancer.* 2010 Jun;17(2):351-60.

56. Memmott RM, Mercado JR, Maier CR, Kawabata S, Fox SD, Dennis PA. Metformin prevents tobacco carcinogen-induced lung tumorigenesis. *Cancer Prev Res (Phila Pa).* 2010 Sep;3(9):1066-76.

57. Faloon W. Consumer rape. *Life Extension Magazine®.* 2002 Apr;8(4).

58. Available at: http://www.cmpi.org/in-the-news/in-the-news/growing-problem-of-fake-drugs-hurting-patients-companies/. Accessed March 25, 2011.

59. Available at: http://www.fda.gov/NewsEvents/Newsroom/PressAnnouncements/ucm242234.htm. Accessed March 25, 2011.

60. Available at: http://www.suntimes.com/lifestyles/health/4230222-423/company-hikes-preemie-preventive-drug-from-10-to-1500.html. Accessed March 28, 2011.

61. Available at: http://www.fda.gov/NewsEvents/Newsroom/PressAnnouncements/ucm242234.htm. Accessed March 25, 2011.

62. Available at: http://articles.latimes.com/2011/apr/01/news/la-pn-makena-price-cut-fda-20110401. Accessed March 28, 2011.

63. Himmelstein DU, Thorne D, Warren E, Woolhandler S. Medical bankruptcy in the United States, 2007: results of a national study. *Am J Med.* 2009 Aug;122(8):741-6.

64. Available at: http://workers-compensation.blogspot.com/2010/11/usps-may-declare-bankruptcy-citing-high.html. Accessed March 28, 2011.

65. Available at: http://www.forbes.com/2009/05/14/taxes-social-security-opinions-columnists-medicare.html. Accessed March 24, 2011.

Preamble

HOW PHARMACEUTICAL INTERESTS MANIPULATE CONGRESS INTO BANKRUPTING OUR HEALTHCARE SYSTEM

BEFORE READING THE REVEALING CHAPTERS in *Pharmocracy*, it is critical to understand the magnitude of control that pharmaceutical and other special interests exert in Washington. The tragic result is that corrupt legislation is enacted that garners outlandish profits to those with political connections, while driving up healthcare costs to levels that are unaffordable by governmental and private entities.

The Medicare Prescription Drug Act is an egregious example of how Congress can be corrupted into passing laws that pour hundreds of billions of dollars in profits into Big Pharma, while hastening the financial collapse of our healthcare system.

For years, Life Extension® fought a brutal battle in an attempt to prevent the Medicare Prescription Drug Act from passing in Congress. This 1,000-page bill, written by pharmaceutical lobbyists, provided $395 billion of taxpayer

subsidies over a ten-year period for the purchase of prescription drugs at full retail prices.[1]

Just imagine you owned a business (like a pharmaceutical
company) in which you sold a product for $100 that cost you
only $5 to make. You are protected against competition by
federal agencies that destroy those who make less expensive
options (like alternative therapies) available. Your only problem is that consumers cannot afford your overpriced product.

Most industries respond to these kinds of issues by initiating more efficient business practices and cutting prices.
What if, instead of lowering prices, you influenced the federal government to use tax dollars to buy your overpriced
product? That's exactly what the pharmaceutical industry
accomplished when they snuck through the Medicare Prescription Drug Act, with more drug lobbyists in the halls of
Congress that night than elected officials.[2]

Here is an excerpt from what was reported by CBS News's
60 Minutes about this bill:

> If you have ever wondered why the costs of pre-
> scription drugs in the United States are the
> highest in the world or why it's illegal to import
> cheaper drugs from Canada or Mexico, you need
> look no further than the pharmaceutical lobby
> and its influence in Washington, DC. According
> to a new report by the Center for Public Integ-
> rity, congressmen are outnumbered two to one
> by lobbyists for an industry that spends roughly
> a $100 million a year in campaign contributions
> and lobbying expenses to protect its profits.[3]

Enacted in 2003, the Medicare Prescription Drug Act
prohibits Medicare from using its enormous purchasing
power to negotiate lower prices.[4] This means taxpayers
are stuck with the tab of paying around 60% more than

government agencies, like the Veteran's Administration, which are allowed to negotiate drug price discounts.[5]

HOW THE DRUG LOBBY WORKS

The full name of this corruptly passed legislation is the Medicare Prescription Drug, Improvement, and Modernization Act.

The insidious way this law was passed provides an intriguing window into how pharmaceutical influence causes Americans to overpay for prescription drugs and then plunders tax dollars to subsidize some of those who cannot afford the artificially inflated prices.

The Medicare Prescription Drug Act was passed at 3:00 am, long after most people in Washington had gone to sleep. Most members of Congress initially refused to vote for the bill, arguing it was too expensive and provided a windfall to the drug companies. The drug lobbyists went into overdrive, going as far as to threaten to support opposing candidates in future elections if certain members of Congress did not vote for the bill.[1, 3, 6]

Despite there being no surplus federal revenue available to fund the Medicare Prescription Drug Act, pharmaceutical lobbying prevailed over ethical consciousness as Congress narrowly enacted this bill.

To add insult to injury, within two weeks of the bill's passage, Medicare released data showing the true projected cost of the bill would be $534 billion, instead of the $395 billion Congress was misled into believing.[7]

In sworn testimony before Congress, it was revealed this $534 billion cost projection was intentionally withheld from Congress on orders from a Medicare official who went to work for a high-powered Washington, DC, lobbying firm ten days after the bill was signed into law.[3, 8, 9]

If these numbers don't appall you, just two years later, in 2005, the White House released revised budgetary figures showing the cost to the US Treasury of the Medicare Prescription Drug Act may have been as high as $1.2 trillion—three times greater than what Congress was misled to believe![10]

Outsiders who helped push through the Medicare Prescription Drug Act included many former members of Congress who were registered lobbyists for the drug industry. Pharmaceutical companies have long been known to reward former members of Congress with lucrative employment contracts.[1, 11–14]

In fact, Billy Tauzin, the congressman most responsible for pushing through the Medicare Prescription Drug Act, retired to a $2 million-a-year job as president of the Pharmaceutical Research and Manufacturers of America.[2] Fourteen other congressional staffers, congressmen, and federal officials also went to work for the pharmaceutical industry after the Medicare Prescription Drug Act was passed—a bill that will pour over one trillion tax (or debt) dollars into drug company coffers.[2, 15]

HIGH PRICE OF CITIZEN APATHY

The squalid facts behind passage of the Medicare Prescription Drug Act leave no doubt as to how much power the drug industry wields over us. While consumer groups like the Life Extension Foundation® tried to defeat this crooked legislation, the sad fact is that too many members of Congress betrayed their constituencies and capitulated to the drug lobbyists.

The Medicare Prescription Drug Act was enacted because the American citizenry remained oblivious to this conspiracy to pillage tax dollars and funnel hundreds of billions of additional profits to the pharmaceutical industry.

In a market free of government regulation, drug prices would collapse in response to competitive pressures. Instead, prescription drug prices remain excruciatingly high. When faced with the prospect of having to lower their prices, the pharmaceutical industry instead perpetrated schemes (like the Medicare Prescription Drug Act) that force virtually every American to subsidize their egregiously overpriced drugs.

If only a small fraction of the American public had voiced their outrage to Congress, the Medicare Prescription Drug Act would not have passed. Now that we know the realities of what this and other shady Medicare/Medicaid programs are really going to cost, each taxpayer faces the prospect of paying thousands of additional Medicare tax dollars every single year. Yet even with higher taxes, Medicare's eventual date with insolvency is inevitable unless medicine is radically deregulated.

This book comprises only a fraction of articles I have written over the past 27 years to expose the charade of medical regulation that is slowly bankrupting our country.

Unlike other books of this nature, I propose real-world solutions that, if implemented, can save this nation from insolvency as it vainly attempts offset the corrosive effects of regulations that breed institutionalized corruption.

As you read the chapters of this book that date back to the 1990s, you will realize how Life Extension's early warnings have manifested into a harsh reality that can no longer be ignored.

References

1. Available at: http://www.publicintegrity.org/hiredguns/. Accessed March 25, 2011.
2. Available at: http://www.citizen.org/congress/article_redirect.cfm?ID=7827. Accessed March 28, 2011.

3. Availableat:www.cbsnews.com/stories/2007/03/29/60minutes/main2625305.shtml. Accessed March 28, 2011.

4. Availableat:http://www.gpo.gov/fdsys/pkg/PLAW-108publ173/pdf/PLAW-108publ173.pdf. Accessed March 28, 2011.

5. Hayes JM, Walczak H, Prochazka A. Comparison of drug regimen costs between the Medicare prescription discount program and other purchasing systems. *JAMA.* 2005 Jul 27;294(4):427-8.

6. Available at: http://www.citizen.org/congress/reform/rx_benefits/drug_benefit/. Accessed March 28, 2011.

7. Available at: http://articles.latimes.com/2004/jan/30/nation/na-medicare30. Accessed March 28, 2011.

8. Available at: http://www.nationalreview.com/articles/210868/cover-costs/deroy-murdock. Accessed March 28, 2011.

9. Available at: http://www.pbs.org/newshour/updates/medicare_03-17-04.html. Accessed March 28, 2011.

10. Available at: http://www.washingtonpost.com/wp-dyn/articles/A9328-2005Feb8.html. Accessed March 28, 2011.

11. Available at: http://www.taxtyranny.ca/images/HTML/Pharmacartel/Articles/DrugCompanies/Articles/drugmakers2.pdf. Accessed March 29, 2011.

12. Available at: http://www.nytimes.com/2004/07/23/technology/23biotech.html). Accessed March 29, 2011.

13. Available at: http://www.nytimes.com/2004/12/16/politics/16drug.html). Accessed March 29, 2011.

14. Available at: http://query.nytimes.com/gst/fullpage.html?res=950DE3D71F3AF930A35751C1A9659C8B63&pagewanted=2. Accessed March 28, 2011.

15. Available at: http://www.truth-out.org/article/medicare-drug-bill-tied-abramoff. Accessed March 28, 2011.

2011

FDA Says Walnuts Are Illegal Drugs

L IFE EXTENSION® HAS PUBLISHED 57 articles that describe the health benefits of walnuts.

Some of this same scientific data was featured on the website of Diamond Foods, Inc., a distributor of packaged walnuts.

Last year the FDA determined that walnuts sold by Diamond Foods cannot be legally marketed because the walnuts "are not generally recognized as safe and effective" for the medical conditions referenced on Diamond Foods' website.

According to the FDA, these walnuts were classified as "drugs" and the "unauthorized health claims" cause them to become "misbranded," thus subjecting them to government "seizure or injunction."

Diamond Foods capitulated and removed statements about the health benefits of walnuts from its website.

Let's take a look at the science supporting the consumption of walnuts to see what the FDA censored . . . and what you can do to stop it in the future!

EATING WALNUTS CUTS HEART DISEASE RISK

Ingesting nuts used to be considered unhealthy because of their high fat content. This misconception has changed over the past 18 years as human studies have revealed sharply reduced incidence of heart disease in those who consume walnuts.[1-12]

Unlike some nuts, walnuts provide a unique blend of polyunsaturated fatty acids (including omega-3s), along with nutrients like gamma-tocopherol that have demonstrated heart health benefits.[13-24]

The March 4, 1993 issue of the *New England Journal of Medicine* published the first clinical study showing significant reductions in dangerous LDL and improvement in the lipoprotein profile in response to moderate consumption of walnuts.[14] Later studies revealed that walnuts improve endothelial function in ways that are independent of cholesterol reduction.[1, 25-27]

One study published by the American Heart Association journal *Circulation* on April 6, 2004, showed a 64% improvement in a measurement of endothelial function when walnuts were substituted for other fats in a Mediterranean diet.[1]

As most Life Extension® members are aware, the underlying cause of atherosclerosis is progressive endothelial dysfunction.[28] Walnuts contain a variety of nutrients including arginine, polyphenols, and omega-3s that support the inner arterial lining and guard against abnormal platelet aggregation.[2,13,29-31] These favorable biological effects explain why walnut consumption confers protection against coronary artery disease.

The US National Library of Medicine database contains no fewer than 35 peer-reviewed published papers supporting a claim that ingesting walnuts improves vascular health and may reduce heart attack risk.

FDA IGNORES THE SCIENCE

The federal agency responsible for protecting the health of the American public views this differently.

In the FDA's warning letter to Diamond Foods, nowhere is there any challenge questioning the science cited by Diamond Foods to support their health claims.

Instead, the FDA's language resembles that of an out-of-control police state where tyranny reins over rationality. To enable you to recognize the absurdity of all of this, I excerpted a few paragraphs from the FDA's warning letter to Diamond Foods as follows:[32]

> Based on our review, we have concluded that your walnut products are in violation of the Federal Food, Drug, and Cosmetic Act (the Act) and the applicable regulations in Title 21, Code of Federal Regulations (21 CFR).
>
> Based on claims made on your firm's website, we have determined that your walnut products are promoted for conditions that cause them to be drugs because these products are intended for use in the prevention, mitigation, and treatment of disease.
>
> Because of these intended uses, your walnut products are drugs within the meaning of section 201 (g)(1)(B) of the Act [21 U.S.C. § 321(g)(B)]. Your walnut products are also new drugs under section 201(p) of the Act [21 U.S.C. § 321(p)] because they are not generally recognized as safe and effective for the above referenced conditions. Therefore, under section 505(a) of the Act [21 U.S.C. § 355(a)], they may not be legally marketed with the above claims in the United States without an approved new drug application.

Additionally, your walnut products are offered for conditions that are not amenable to self-diagnosis and treatment by individuals who are not medical practitioners; therefore, adequate directions for use cannot be written so that a layperson can use these drugs safely for their intended purposes. Thus, your walnut products are also misbranded under section 502(f)(1) of the Act, in that the labeling for these drugs fails to bear adequate directions for use [21 U.S.C. § 352(f)(1)].

This verbiage makes it clear that the FDA does not even consider the underlying science when censoring truthful, non-misleading health claims. The chilling effect on the ability of consumers to discover lifesaving medical information is a wake-up call for all who recognize the ramifications of this latest act of FDA malfeasance.

WHAT THE FDA ALLOWS YOU TO HEAR

The number of people logging on to the website of Diamond Foods was miniscule. I suspect that before the FDA took this draconian action, hardly anyone even knew this website existed.

What the public hears loud and clear, however, are endless advertisements for artery-clogging junk foods. Fast food chains relentlessly promote their 99-cent double-cheese burger as being bigger than their rivals. These advertisements induce many consumers to salivate for these toxic calories that are a contributing cause of coronary artery disease. Yet the FDA does not utter a peep in suggesting that their advertising be curtailed.

On the contrary, FDA has issued waves of warning letters to companies making foods (pomegranate juice, green tea, and walnuts) that protect against atherosclerosis.[1,32-36] The FDA is blatantly demanding that these companies stop informing the public about the scientifically validated health benefits these foods provide.

The FDA obviously does not want the public to discover that they can reduce their risk of age-related disease by consuming healthy foods. They prefer consumers only learn about mass-marketed garbage foods that shorten life span by increasing degenerative disease risk.

FDA ALLOWS POTATO CHIPS TO BE ADVERTISED AS "HEART HEALTHY"

Frito-Lay® is a subsidiary of the PepsiCo, Inc., makers of Pepsi cola. Frito-Lay® sells $12 billion a year of products that include:

- Lays® Potato Chips
- Doritos®
- Tostitos®
- Cheetos®
- Fritos®

You might not associate these mostly-fried snack foods as being good for you, but the FDA has no problem allowing the Frito-Lay® website to state the following:

> Frito-Lay® snacks start with real farm-grown ingredients. You might be surprised at how much good stuff goes into your favorite snack. Good stuff like potatoes, which naturally contain vitamin C and essential minerals. Or corn, one of the world's most popular grains, packed with thiamin, vitamin B6, and phosphorous—all necessary for healthy bones, teeth, nerves and muscles.

And it's not just the obvious ingredients. Our all-natural sunflower, corn and soybean oils contain good polyunsaturated and monounsaturated fats, which help lower total and LDL "bad" cholesterol and maintain HDL "good" cholesterol levels, which can support a healthy heart. Even salt, when eaten in moderation as part of a balanced diet, is essential for the body.[37]

Wow! Based on what Frito-Lay® is allowed to state, it sounds like we should be living on these snacks. Who would want to ingest walnuts, pomegranate, or green tea (which the FDA is now attacking) when these fat calorie-laden, mostly-fried carbohydrates are so widely available?

According to the Frito Lay® website, Lays® potato chips are now "heart healthy" because the level of saturated fat was reduced and replaced with sunflower oil.[38] Scientific studies do show that when a polyunsaturated fat (like sunflower oil) is substituted for saturated fat, favorable changes in blood cholesterol occur.[39]

Fatally omitted from the Frito-Lay® website is the fact that sunflower oil supplies lots of omega-6 fats, but no omega-3s.[40] The American diet already contains too many omega-6 fats and woefully inadequate omega-3s.

Excess omega-6 fats in the diet in the absence of adequate omega-3s produces devastating effects, including the production of pro-inflammatory compounds that contribute to virtually every age-related disease, including atherosclerosis.[41-45]

For the FDA to allow Frito-Lay® to pretend there are heart benefits to ingesting their unhealthy snack products, while censoring the ability of walnut companies to make scientifically substantiated claims, is tantamount to treason against the health of the American public.

DON'T FORGET THE ACRYLAMIDES

When carbohydrate foods are cooked at high temperature (as occurs when potatoes are fried in sunflower oil to make potato chips), a toxic compound called arcylamide is formed.[46]

According to the National Cancer Institute, "acrylamide is considered to be a mutagen and a probable human carcinogen, based mainly on studies in laboratory animals. Scientists do not yet know with any certainty whether the levels of acrylamide typically found in some foods pose a health risk for humans."[47]

In response to these kinds of concerns, the FDA funded a massive study to ascertain the acrylamide content of various foods. The FDA found that potato chips and other fried carbohydrate foods were especially high in acrylamides.[48]

The FDA, however, has not stopped companies selling high acrylamide-containing fried carbohydrates from promoting these foods as healthy.

PHARMACEUTICAL COMPANIES BENEFIT FROM FDA'S MISDEEDS

As the aging population develops coronary atherosclerosis, pharmaceutical companies stand to reap tens of billions of dollars each year in profits. An obstacle standing in their way is scientific evidence showing that a healthy diet can prevent heart disease from developing in many people.

It is thus in the economic interests of pharmaceutical giants that the FDA forcibly censor the ability of companies making heart healthy foods to inform the public of the underlying science. The fewer consumers who know the facts about walnuts, pomegranate, and green tea, the greater the demand will be for expensive cardiac drugs.

Once again, the FDA overtly functions to enrich Big Pharma, while the public shoulders the financial burden of today's healthcare cost crisis.

In this particular case, however, processed food companies also stand to profit from the FDA's attacks on healthy foods.

CHILLING EFFECT ON INNOVATION

Headquartered in Stockton, California, Diamond Foods is a processor and marketer of nuts, with distribution in over 80% of US supermarkets. Most of Diamond's 1,700 walnut growers are family farmers with orchards in the heartland of California's Central Valley. Their association with Diamond guarantees a market for their crops and provides the company with high-quality walnuts.

In response to independent scientific studies validating the health benefits of walnuts, Diamond Foods made financial investments to educate the public and supply them with walnuts. With one misguided letter issued by the FDA, all of Diamond Foods good work was undone.

This kind of bureaucratic tyranny sends a strong signal to the food industry not to innovate in a way that informs the public about foods that protect against disease. While consumers increasingly reach for healthier dietary choices, the federal government wants to deny food companies the ability to convey findings from scientific studies about their products.

FDA/FTC WANTS MORE CONTROL OVER WHAT YOU ARE ALLOWED TO LEARN

The FDA and FTC (Federal Trade Commission) are proposing new regulations that will stifle the ability of natural food companies to disseminate scientific research findings.

One proposal being discussed within the FTC would require that supplement companies conduct studies analogous to what the FDA requires to approve new drugs. In a perfect world, Life Extension® would agree with some of the FTC's objectives. As far as we are concerned, the more scientific research to validate a health claim, the better.

The reality is that natural foods do not carry high prescription drug price markups, so it would be economically impossible to conduct the same kinds of voluminous clinical studies as pharmaceutical companies do. As readers of this column know, many of the clinical studies the FDA relies on to approve new drugs are fraudulent to begin with. So even if it were feasible to conduct more clinical research on foods and supplements, that still does not guarantee the precise accuracy the FTC is seeking.

If these agency proposals are enacted, consumers will be barred from learning about new ways to protect their health until a food or nutrient meets stringent new requirements. A look at the warning letter the FDA sent to Diamond Foods is a frightening example of how scientific information can be harshly censored by unelected bureaucrats.

If anyone still thinks that federal agencies like the FDA protect the public, this latest proclamation that healthy foods are now illegal drugs exposes the government's sordid charade.

COMPANIES THAT SELL HEALTHY FOODS TRY TO FIGHT BACK

The combined sales of the companies attacked by the FDA are only a fraction of those of food giant Frito-Lay®. Yet some of these companies are fighting back against the FDA's absurd position that it is illegal to disseminate scientific research showing the favorable effects these foods produce in the body. The makers of pomegranate juice, for example, have sued the FTC for censoring their First Amendment right to communicate scientific information to the public.

As a consumer, you should be outraged that disease-promoting foods are protected by the federal government, while nutritious foods are censored. There is no scientific rationale for the FDA to do this. On the contrary, the dangerous foods ubiquitously advertised in the media are replacing cigarettes as the leading killers in modern society.

The federal government is heavily lobbied by companies selling processed foods. As Life Extension® revealed long ago, an insidious activity of lobbyists is to incite federal agencies and prosecutors to eliminate free competition in the marketplace.

The simple fact is that walnuts are healthy to eat, while carbohydrates fried in fat are not. The FDA permits companies selling disease-promoting foods to deceive the public, while it suppresses the dissemination of peer-reviewed published scientific information.

NOW THE GOOD NEWS . . .

On April 5, 2011, a bipartisan bill was introduced into the House of Representatives called the Free Speech about Science Act (H.R. 1364). This landmark legislation protects basic free speech rights, ends censorship of science, and enables the natural health products community to share peer-reviewed scientific findings with the public.

The Free Speech about Science bill has the potential to transform medical practice by educating the public about the real science behind natural health.

For this very reason, the bill will have opposition. It will be opposed by the FDA since it restricts their ability to censor the dissemination of published scientific data. It will be opposed by drug companies fearing competition from natural health approaches based on diet, dietary supplements, and lifestyle.

The public, on the other hand, wants access to credible information they can use to make wise dietary choices. Please don't let special interests stop this bill.

I ask readers of this book to log on to our Legislative Action Website (www.lef.org/lac) that enables you to conveniently email and ask your Representative to cosponsor the Free Speech about Science Act (H.R. 1364).

Passage of the Free Speech about Science Act will stop federal agencies from squandering tax dollars censoring what you are allowed to learn about health-promoting foods.

Our Legislative Action Website provides you direct contact with your Representative to let them know that you want H.R. 1364 (Free Speech about Science Act) enacted into law.

This same website lets you send the Introduction of this book to your Representative and two Senators along with a form letter to encourage Congress to enact legislation to remove the regulatory stranglehold over healthcare that is rendering this nation insolvent.

> When the people fear their government, there is tyranny; when the government fears the people, there is liberty.
>
> —THOMAS JEFFERSON

References

1. Ros E, Nunez I, Perez-Heras A, et al. A walnut diet improves endothelial function in hypercholesterolemic subjects: a randomized crossover trial. *Circulation*. 2004 Apr 6;109(13):1609–14.

2. Feldman EB. The scientific evidence for a beneficial health relationship between walnuts and coronary heart disease. *J Nutr*. 2002 May;132(5):1062S–1101S.

3. Blomhoff R, Carlsen MH, Andersen LF, Jacobs DR Jr. Health benefits of nuts: potential role of antioxidants. *Br J Nutr*. 2006 Nov;96 Suppl 2:S52–60.

4. Mozaffarian D. Does alpha-linolenic acid intake reduce the risk of coronary heart disease? A review of the evidence. *Altern Ther Health Med*. 2005 May-Jun;11(3):24–30; quiz 31, 79.

5. Zhao G, Etherton TD, Martin KR, West SG, Gillies PJ, Kris-Etherton PM. Dietary alpha-linolenic acid reduces inflammatory and lipid cardiovascular risk factors in hypercholesterolemic men and women. *J Nutr*. 2004 Nov;134(11):2991–7.

6. Tapsell LC, Gillen LJ, Patch CS, Batterham M, Owen A, Baré M, Kennedy M. Including walnuts in a low-fat/modified-fat diet improves HDL cholesterol-to-total cholesterol ratios in patients with type 2 diabetes. *Diabetes Care*. 2004 Dec;27(12):2777–83.

7. West SG, Boseka L, Wagner P. Alpha-linolenic acid from walnuts and flax increases flow-mediated dilation of the brachial artery in a dose-dependent fashion. Poster presented at the American Heart Association's 5th Annual Conference on Arteriosclerosis, Thrombosis, and Vascular Biology. San Francisco, CA: May 6, 2004.

8. Iwamoto M, Imaizumi K, Sato M, Hirooka Y, Sakai K, Takeshita A, Kono M. Serum lipid profiles in Japanese women and men during consumption of walnuts. *Eur JClin Nutr*. 2002 Jul;56(7):629–37.

9. Morgan JM, Horton K, Reese D, et al. Effects of walnut consumption as part of a low-fat, low-cholesterol diet on serum cardiovascular risk factors. *Int J Vit Nutr Research*. 2002 Oct;72(5):341–7.

10. Hu FB, Stampfer MJ, Manson JE, et al. Frequent nut consumption and risk of coronary heart disease in women: prospective cohort study. *BMJ*. 1998 Nov 14;317(7169):1341–5.

11. Chisholm A, Mann J, Skeaff M, et al. A diet rich in walnuts favourably influences plasma fatty acid profile in moderately hyperlipidaemic subjects. *Eur J Clin Nutr*. 1998 Jan;52(1):12–6.

12. de Lorgeril M, Renaud S, Mamelle N, et al. Mediterranean alpha-linolenic acid-rich diet in secondary prevention of coronary heart disease. *Lancet*. 1994 Jun 11;343(8911):1454–9.

13. Maguire LS, O'Sullivan SM, Galvin K, O'Connor TP, O'Brien NM. Fatty acid profile, tocopherol, squalene and phytosterol content of walnuts, almonds, peanuts, hazelnuts and the macadamia nut. *Int J Food Sci Nutr*. 2004 May;55(3):171–8.

14. Sabate J, Fraser GE, Burke K, Knutsen SF, Bennett H, Lindsted KD. Effects of walnuts on serum lipid levels and blood pressure in normal men. *N Engl J Med*. 1993 Mar 4;328(9):603–7.

15. Zambon D, Sabate J, Munoz S, et al. Substituting walnuts for monounsaturated fat improves the serum lipid profile of hypercholesterolemic men and women. A randomized crossover trial. *Ann Intern Med*. 2000 Apr 4;132(7):538–46.

16. Iwamoto M, Imaizumi K, Sato M, et al. Serum lipid profiles in Japanese women and men during consumption of walnuts. *Eur J Clin Nutr*. 2002 Jul;56(7):629–37.

17. Simopoulos AP. Essential fatty acids in health and chronic disease. *Am J Clin Nutr*. 1999 Sep;70(3 Suppl):560S–569S.

18. Hu FB, Stampfer MJ. Nut consumption and risk of coronary heart disease: a review of epidemiologic evidence. *Curr Atheroscler Rep*. 1999 Nov;1(3):204–9.

19. Zibaeenezhad MJ, Rezaiezadeh M, Mowla A, Ayatollahi SM, Panjehshahin MR. Antihypertriglyceridemic effect of walnut oil. *Angiology*. 2003 Jul-Aug;54(4):411–4.

20. Almario RU, Vonghavaravat V, Wong R, Kasim-Karakas SE. Effects of walnut consumption on plasma fatty acids and lipoproteins in combined hyperlipidemia. *Am J Clin Nutr*. 2001 Jul;74(1):72–9.

21. Anderson KJ, Teuber SS, Gobeille A, Cremin P, Waterhouse AL, Steinberg FM. Walnut polyphenolics inhibit in vitro human plasma and LDL oxidation. *J Nutr*. 2001 Nov;131(11):2837–42.

22. Singh I, Turner AH, Sinclair AJ, Li D, Hawley JA. Effects of gamma-tocopherol supplementation on thrombotic risk factors. *Asia Pac J Clin Nutr*. 2007;16(3):422–8.

23. McCarty MF. Gamma-tocopherol may promote effective no synthase function by protecting tetrahydrobiopterin from peroxynitrite. *Med Hypotheses*. 2007;69(6):1367–70.

24. Park SK, Page GP, Kim K, et al. alpha- and gamma-Tocopherol prevent age-related transcriptional alterations in the heart and brain of mice. *J Nutr*. 2008 Jun;138(6):1010–8.

25. Cortés B, Núñez I, Cofán M, et al. Acute effects of high-fat meals enriched with walnuts or olive oil on postprandial endothelial function. *J Am Coll Cardiol*. 2006 Oct 17;48(8):1666–71.

26. Ros E, Mataix J. Fatty acid composition of nuts—implications for cardiovascular health. *Br J Nutr*. 2006 Nov;96 Suppl 2:S29–35.

27. Ma Y, Njike VY, Millet J, et al. Effects of walnut consumption on endothelial function in type 2 diabetic subjects: a randomized controlled crossover trial. *Diabetes Care*. 2010 Feb;33(2):227–32.

28. Le Brocq M, Leslie SJ, Milliken P, Megson IL. Endothelial dysfunction: from molecular mechanisms to measurement, clinical implications, and therapeutic opportunities. *Antioxid Redox Signal*. 2008 Sep;10(9):1631–74.

29. Ros E. Nuts and novel biomarkers of cardiovascular disease. *Am J Clin Nutr*. 2009 May;89(5):1649S–56S.

30. Feldman EB. The scientific evidence for a beneficial health relationship between walnuts and coronary heart disease. *J Nutr*. 2002 May;132(5):1062S–1101S.

31. Ristic-Medic D, Ristic G, Tepsic V. Alpha-linolenic acid and cardiovascular diseases. *Med Pregl*. 2003;56 Suppl 1:19–25.

32. Available at: http://www.fda.gov/ICECI/EnforcementActions/WarningLetters/ucm202825.htm. Accessed March 26, 2010.

33. Aviram M, Rosenblat M, Gaitini D, et al. Pomegranate juice consumption for 3 years by patients with carotid artery stenosis reduces common carotid intima-media thickness, blood pressure and LDL oxidation. *Clin Nutr.* 2004 Jun;23(3):423–33.

34. Oyama J, Maeda T, Kouzuma K, et al. Green tea catechins improve human forearm endothelial dysfunction and have antiatherosclerotic effects in smokers. *Circ J.* 2010 Mar;74(3):578–88.

35. Available at: http://www.fda.gov/ICECI/EnforcementActions/WarningLetters/ucm202785.htm. Accessed April 11, 2011.

36. Available at: http://www.fda.gov/ICECI/EnforcementActions/WarningLetters/ucm224509.htm. Accessed April 11, 2011.

37. Available at: http://www.fritolay.com/your-health/whats-in-our-snacks.html. Accessed March 25, 2010.

38. Available at: http://www.fritolay.com/about-us/press-release-20060503.html. March 25, 2010.

39. Jakobsen MU, O'Reilly EJ, Heitmann BL, et al. Major types of dietary fat and risk of coronary heart disease: a pooled analysis of 11 cohort studies. *Am J Clin Nutr.* 2009 May;89(5):1425–32.

40. Scherr C, Ribeiro JP. Fat content of dairy products, eggs, margarines and oils: implications for atherosclerosis. *Arq Bras Cardiol.* 2010 Jul;95(1):55–60.

41. Available at: http://www.kedu.us/Ask%20the%20Doctor/omega%203%20cardiovascular.pdf. Accessed March 29, 2010.

42. Simopoulos AP. The importance of the omega-6/omega-3 fatty acid ratio in cardiovascular disease and other chronic diseases. *Exp Biol Med* (Maywood). 2008 Jun;233(6):674–88.

43. Okuyama H, Kobayashi T, Watanabe S. Dietary fatty acids— the N-6/N-3 balance and chronic elderly diseases. Excess linoleic acid and relative N-3 deficiency syndrome seen in Japan. *Prog Lipid Res.* 1996 Dec;35(4):409–57.

44. Kiecolt-Glaser JK, Belury MA, Porter K, et al. Depressive symptoms, omega-6:omega-3 fatty acids, and inflammation in older adults. *Psychosom Med.* 2007 Apr;69(3):217–24.

45. Guebre-Egziabher F, Rabasa-Lhoret R, Bonnet F, et al. Nutritional intervention to reduce the n-6/n-3 fatty acid ratio

increases adiponectin concentration and fatty acid oxidation in healthy subjects. *Eur J Clin Nutr.* 2008 Nov;62(11):1287-93.

46. Jackson LS, Al-Taher F. Effects of consumer food preparation on acrylamide formation. *Adv Exp Med Biol.* 2005 561:447-65.

47. Available at: http://www.cancer.gov/cancertopics/factsheet/Risk/Fs3_96.pdf. Accessed April 11, 2010.

48. Available at: http://www.fda.gov/food/foodsafety/foodcontaminantsadulteration/chemicalcontaminants/acrylamide/ucm053569.htm. Accessed April 11, 2011.

The FDA's Most Heinous Drug Approval

W HEN IT COMES to lethal FDA-approved drugs, I always felt that Life Extension® members had a better chance of surviving adverse reactions compared to the general public.

One reason is that members have their blood tested annually so they can detect many types of drug toxicities before permanent damage is inflicted. Another defense members have are the healthy lifestyles they follow, which confers protection against mechanisms by which prescription drugs kill, such as glutathione depletion and fatty acid metabolite imbalance.[1-5]

When it comes to the fraudulent drug you are about to read about, however, it would have been challenging for any of us to survive. This deadly drug was administered intravenously during complex surgical procedures when one's life is completely at the mercy of others.

I am going to relate what may be the most atrocious cover-up of a toxic drug that a pharmaceutical company has ever perpetrated—a drug that the FDA should have never approved.

WHY SOME SURGERY PATIENTS NEED THESE KINDS OF DRUGS

A common surgical complication is excessive bleeding. In patients with a high risk of bleeding, intravenous drugs are administered ahead of time.

While lower-cost alternative drugs are available to reduce bleeding complications, pharmaceutical giant Bayer penetrated the market with a drug called Trasylol® that costs about $1,000 per patient.

If you wonder how this price gouging occurs, large drug companies aggressively promote expensive new drugs to doctors, in some cases paying cash kickbacks so that the more expensive drug is used in place of an alternative of equal efficacy.

In the case of Trasylol®, the results turned tragic.

THE FDA'S ERRONEOUS APPROVAL OF TRASYLOL®

Despite data showing that Trasylol® inflicted severe kidney damage in animals,[6] the FDA approved it for human use in 1993.[7] Low-cost alternative anti-bleeding drugs are less likely to produce this lethal side effect.

Soon, the same kidney side effects observed in animals were occurring in humans. One surgeon observed that the most common side effect seen in patients given Trasylol® was renal dysfunction. This surgeon then conducted a 20-patient study (not funded by Bayer) and found that 13 of 20 patients given Trasylol® had problems with kidney function after the surgical procedure.[8]

When the FDA approved Trasylol®, they did note that kidney toxicity was a problem. But Bayer lobbied the FDA hard and by 1998, the FDA expanded approval of Trasylol® to cover all heart bypass patients.[9]

Sales of Trasylol® in 2005 hit $300 million and Bayer envisioned a billion-dollar-per-year blockbuster.[10] These kinds of profits provide an enormous war chest to lobby FDA officials to turn a blind eye, even while thousands of surgical patients were dying each year from kidney failure caused by Trasylol®.

Investigators were initially perplexed because kidney toxicity showed up in some studies, but not others. Critics maintain that Bayer never paid for studies large enough to determine the renal toxicity of Trasylol®.

The primary side effect mechanism of Trasylol® is that it causes excess blood clotting inside blood vessels (thrombosis).[11] This made tissues throughout the body vulnerable to loss of blood flow, which is why patients given Trasylol® sometimes died from multiple organ failure—plus amputation of limbs.

TRASYLOL® CARNAGE COVERED UP BY BAYER

In 2006, a study was released showing that thousands of Americans were being killed each year by Trasylol®.[11] The FDA responded by issuing an "advisory" alerting doctors to this potential problem, but did not plan to have a formal meeting about Trasylol® for eight months.[12, 13]

Bayer was desperate to keep Trasylol® on the market, so it hired a respected Harvard professor to look at the records of nearly 70,000 patients treated with Trasylol®. The Harvard professor's report did not please Bayer. It revealed that horrific numbers of Americans had died from Trasylol®. The Harvard professor wrote that patients on Trasylol® had an elevated risk of death and acute kidney failure.[10]

When the FDA finally held an advisory committee meeting to address the Trasylol® deaths, Bayer intentionally *withheld* the Harvard professor's exhaustive study.[14] Since the FDA did not know of Bayer's negative study, it voted to keep Trasylol® on the market.

A week later, the Harvard professor went to the FDA to inform them that Bayer had hidden the study showing the lethal dangers of Trasylol®.[15] The FDA's response was to issue another warning to doctors.[16] Bayer meanwhile continued to sell hundreds of millions of dollars worth of Trasylol® to unsuspecting surgical patients.

ONE THOUSAND LIVES LOST EACH MONTH BECAUSE OF THE FDA'S DELAY IN REMOVING TRASYLOL®

In 2007, the Canadian government terminated a study using Trasylol® because too many patients were dying.[17] Germany responded to this study by banning Trasylol® altogether.[18] The FDA's initial response was to convince Bayer to suspend marketing of Trasylol® only temporarily.[19, 20]

In 2008, amid a flurry of lawsuits, Bayer announced that it was removing the remaining supply of Trasylol® from the American market.[21]

Experts estimate that had the FDA taken action when the first report came out, 22,000 lives could have been saved—which equates to about 1,000 needless deaths each month the FDA failed to act.[10]

Bayer suspended two employees[22] for failing to disclose the Harvard study to the FDA. As with other pharmaceutical companies that cover up the lethal dangers of their drugs, the FDA has taken no action against Bayer. Contrast FDA inaction against Bayer to FDA's threats to imprison growers of cherries and walnuts for promoting the health benefits of their foods.[23, 24]

This kind of unconscionable overcharging is just one of many reasons why our sick-care system is collapsing into a financial abyss.

NOW THAT TRASYLOL® IS GONE . . .
ALTERNATIVE DRUG PRICES SKYROCKET

When CBS News first broke this story, they stated that safer drugs that effectively reduced bleeding complications cost only around $50.00 (compared to around $1,000 for Trasylol®).[10]

Now that Trasylol® has been removed from the market, alternative drugs (such as aminocaproic acid) cost around $750 per surgical procedure based on information that took us months to extract from hospitals. No hospital wanted to volunteer what they charge for aminocaproic acid. This may be because of the absurd price-gouging that routinely occurs at hospital pharmacies, such as charging $10 for an aspirin tablet.

WHY HEALTHCARE COSTS SO MUCH

The side effects attributed to Trasylol® include heart attack, stroke, and kidney failure, as well as excruciating slow deaths.[25]

The medical costs of caring for patients injured by Trasylol® are incomprehensible. In some cases, relatively healthy people suffered so much tissue damage that they were hospitalized in ICU units for months before they died. Other victims required thrice-weekly kidney dialysis, kidney transplants, lifetime nursing home care, and numerous other medical costs, not to mention lost productivity.[26, 27]

If you ever wonder why medical costs are bankrupting the United States, look no further than the fraudulently approved drugs that permeate the marketplace. When government-approved medicines inflict this kind of carnage, the inevitable result is an explosive growth in the numbers of Americans requiring expensive chronic healthcare.

FEDERAL GOVERNMENT DOES NOT PROTECT US

On April 2, 2010, CNN published an article titled, "Fed found Pfizer too big to nail." It described in detail the criminal activities perpetrated to illegally market the drug Bextra® to treat surgical pain and how Federal authorities allowed a subsidiary to plead guilty to the fraud to avoid the harsh sanctions that Pfizer would otherwise face. Such sanctions would have meant that Pfizer would have been excluded from lucrative Medicare and Medicaid payments.

Like other drugs in the COX-2 inhibitor class, Bextra® was shown to increase heart attack risk and was withdrawn from the market.[28] The unfortunate consequence for many surgical patients, however, is that they were exposed to two lethal drugs (Trasylol® and Bextra®) at a time when these patients were particularly vulnerable to pathological clotting inside blood vessels (thrombosis).

Trasylol® was first administered intravenously to prevent excess bleeding, but in reality caused excess blood clotting inside the arteries of many of its victims.[29] In the post-surgical setting, patients were sometimes prescribed a double dose of Bextra® to alleviate surgical pain. One pathological effect of Bextra® is to increase a fatty acid metabolite called thromboxane A2 which further increases thrombotic risk.[4, 5] If you wonder why so many hospital patients die from "surgical complications," look no further than the FDA-approved drugs they were given.

Trasylol® was allowed to remain on the market for 14 years, whereas Bextra® was illegally touted for less than 5 years before being withdrawn.[30] Life Extension® warned about the dangers of drugs like Bextra® and Vioxx® within a year of the FDA approving them.[31] We were in the dark about Trasylol®, however, since this was a drug that surgeons made a decision on using.

The bottom line is that prescription drug costs are contributing to the bankruptcy of this nation's healthcare system. Yet the federal government continues to deceive consumers into believing that they must pay inflated costs in order to be assured of safety and efficacy.

The reality is that high costs give pharmaceutical companies enormous profits that they use to fraudulently promote their drugs, pay off doctors, and lobby both the FDA and Congress to protect their stranglehold over which drugs consumers have access to.[32-34]

Life Extension® remains committed to protecting its members against the blatant corruption that exists today between pharmaceutical companies that engage in fraud to promote dangerous drugs and the politicians and bureaucrats who allow this murderous conspiracy to perpetuate.

BLOOD TESTS CAN DETECT DRUG TOXICITIES IN TIME TO REVERSE DAMAGE

Blood tests that evaluate liver, kidney, muscle, and bone marrow function can detect a wide range of drug toxicities long before permanent damage occurs.

For instance, if a blood test finding uncovers specific tissue damage, a careful evaluation of the drugs you are taking can pinpoint the one causing the problem so you can discontinue it. This usually reverses the damage. Failure to catch a drug-induced pathology in time can result in irreversible system failure.

Regular blood testing can also enable your doctor to adjust the dose of drugs you are taking, and enable you to change your nutrient dose in order to obtain better and safer results.

For example, doctors often prescribe the same dose of a statin drug to every patient. The problem is that the appropriate dose of statin drugs required varies considerably amongst patients. Some can take a small dose (10 mg/day) of a drug like simvastatin and achieve LDL levels below 80 mg/dL, whereas others require higher doses (in addition to nutritional interventions).

Comprehensive blood tests function as a "report card" to verify that the medications, hormones, and supplements you take each day are providing the desired benefits and not inflicting side effects.

When it comes to over-the-counter (OTC) drug toxicity, we at Life Extension® have uncovered it in people as young as 21 years old and reversed it by getting them off daily high-dose analgesics like ibuprofen.

Annual blood testing saves lives not only by detecting drug toxicities, but also revealing vascular risk factors such as elevated triglycerides, glucose, C-reactive protein, and LDL in time to take corrective actions. Hormone imbalances can also be uncovered by proper blood testing and provide a roadmap to enable critical hormones to be safely restored to youthful ranges.

> To inquire about low cost blood testing in your area, call 1-800-208-3444.

P.S. If you want to view the televised report that CBS News did on the Trasylol® travesty, just go to Google and type in: "Trasylol® and 60 Minutes."

References

1. Available at: http://www.mefmaction.net/MECFSFM/Articles/ Treatment/GlutathioneDeficiency/tabid/236/Default.aspx. Accessed November 25, 2010.

2. Available at: http://www.chiro.org/nutrition/FULL/ Recognizing_Drug_Induced_Nutrient_Depletion.shtml. Accessed November 25, 2010.

3. Jaeschke H, Bajt ML. Intracellular signaling mechanisms of acetaminophen-induced liver cell death. *Toxicol Sci.* 2006 Jan;89(1):31–41.

4. Fitzgerald GA. Coxibs and cardiovascular disease. *N Engl J Med.* 2004 Oct 21;351(17):1709–11.

5. Oates JA, FitzGerald GA, Branch RA, Jackson EK, Knapp HR, Roberts LJ 2nd. Clinical implications of prostaglandin and thromboxane A2 formation (1). *N Engl J Med.* 1988 Sep 15;319(11):689–98.

6. Fischer JH, Knupfer P. High-dosage aprotinin (Trasylol) therapy—is it safe for the kidney? *Langenbecks Arch Chir.* 1983;360(4):241–9.

7. Available at: http://www.fda.gov/Drugs/DrugSafety/ PostmarketDrugSafetyInformationforPatientsandProviders/ ucm142740.htm. Accessed March 15, 2011.

8. Sundt TM 3rd, Kouchoukos NT, Saffitz JE, Murphy SF, Wareing TH, Stahl DJ. Renal dysfunction and intravascular coagulation with aprotinin and hypothermic circulatory arrest. *Ann Thorac Surg.* 1993 Jun;55(6):1418–24.

9. Mangano DT, Miao Y, Vuylsteke A, et al. Mortality associated with aprotinin during 5 years following coronary artery bypass graft surgery. *JAMA.* 2007 Feb 7;297(5):471–9.

10. Available at: http://www.cbsnews.com/stories/2008/02/14/ 60minutes/main3831900.shtml. Accessed December 6, 2010.

11. Mangano DT, Tudor IC, Dietzel C; Multicenter Study of Perioperative Ischemia Research Group; Ischemia Research and Education Foundation. The risk associated with aprotinin in cardiac surgery. *N Engl J Med.* 2006 Jan 26;354(4):353–65.

12. Available at: http://www.fda.gov/NewsEvents/Newsroom/ PressAnnouncements/2006/ucm108592.htm. Accessed November 30, 2010.

13. Available at: http://www.investor.bayer.de/en/news/archive/ investor-news-2006/investor news/showNewsItem/669/117 0082441/9c4ca18b75/. Accessed November 30, 2010.

14. Available at: http://www.investor.bayer.de/en/news/ archive/investor-news-2006/investor-news/showNews-Item/673/1168957317/5620356922/. Accessed November 30, 2010.

15. Available at: http://www.corpwatch.org/article.php?id=14185. Accessed December 2, 2010.

16. Available at: http://www.fda.gov/Drugs/DrugSafety/ PostmarketDrugSafetyInformationforPatientsandProviders/ ucm142736.htm. Accessed December 2, 2010.

17. Available at: http://www.washingtonpost.com/wp-dyn/content/ article/2008/05/14/AR2008051401658.html. Accessed December 2, 2010.

18. Available at: http://www.bayer.ca/files/Trasylol,%20BART,%20 November%205,%20FINAL,%20Release.pdf. Accessed December 2, 2010.

19. Available at: http://www.investor.bayer.de/en/news/archive/ investor-news-2007/investor-news/showNewsItem/868/120 1512120/450afb010b. Accessed December 2, 2010.

20. Available at: http://www.fda.gov/downloads/NewsEvents/ Newsroom/MediaTranscripts/UCM122284.pdf. Accessed December 2, 2010.

21. Available at: http://www.consumeraffairs.com/news04/2008/05/ fda_trayslol.html. Accessed December 6, 2010.

22. Available at: http://articles.latimes.com/2006/oct/14/business/ fi-bayer14. Accessed March 15, 2011.

23. Faloon W. FDA threatens to raid cherry orchards. *Life Extension Magazine®*. 2006 Mar;12(3):7–11.

24. Faloon W. FDA says walnuts are illegal drugs. *Life Extension Magazine®*. Publication pending.

25. Available at: http://www.drugwatch.com/trasylol/side-effects. php. Accessed December 6, 2010.

26. Available at: http://www.fda-reports.com/Trasylol.html. Accessed December 9, 2010.

27. Available at: http://www.adrugrecall.com/trasylol/kidney-failure.html. Accessed December 10, 2010.

28. Available at: http://doublecheckmd.com/EffectsDetail.do?dname =Trasylol&sid=1439&eid=3076. Accessed December 10, 2010.

29. Available at: http://www.kcrlegal.com/trasylol.aspx. Accessed December 13, 2010.

30. Available at: http://arthritis.webmd.com/news/20050407/ bextra-taken-off-market-celebrex-gets-warning. Accessed December 15, 2010.

31. Medications side effects. *Life Extension Magazine®*. 2003 Mar.

32. Available at: http://www.naturalnews.com/030111_drug_companies_illegal.html. Accessed December 17, 2010

33. Loewenberg S. US FDA feels the heat from Congressional hearings. *Lancet*. 2008 May 10;371(9624):1565–6.

34. Available at: http://projects.publicintegrity.org/rx/report. aspx?aid=723. Accessed December 17, 2010.

No Real Healthcare Cost Crisis

FOR 31 YEARS LIFE EXTENSION® has warned that corrupt disease-care legislation combined with suffocating FDA regulation will bankrupt the United States of America. The day of reckoning is rapidly approaching when the federal government will be unable to subsidize the hyper-inflated healthcare prices that it created.

We have shown how inefficient and fraudulent government edicts are the cause of today's medical cost crisis—and how this catastrophe can be averted with common-sense changes to the law.[1-3]

A REAL-WORLD EXAMPLE

Life Extension® is on the front lines seven days a week helping people who confront medical issues, many of whom are unable to pay the artificially inflated prices brought on by failed government policies.

I recently received a call from a friend whose younger sister contracted genital herpes and suffered frequent painful outbreaks. Herpes is an incurable virus that 20% of American women (ages 14–49) are infected with.[4] It is estimated that 80% of cases remain undiagnosed.[5]

I suggested that my friend's sister consider taking 500 mg a day of valacyclovir (Valtrex®), as this has been shown to reduce both the number of herpes outbreaks[5] and reduce the chances of spreading the virus to one's sexual partner by 47%.[5] I recalled the retail price of Valtrex® was around $3 per tablet, but thought that it might be available as a lower-priced generic.

When I called the Life Extension® Pharmacy®, I was shocked to learn that the brand-name Valtrex® had jumped to $7.40 per tablet and that the generic cost almost this much! Since Valtrex® needs to be taken every day for prevention of outbreaks, the monthly cost for the generic comes to around $200, bringing the annual price tag to $2,400.

I was outraged that an off-patent drug could be priced this high and ordered our staff to find out what it really cost to produce high-quality generic Valtrex® tablets. What we discovered is beyond abhorrent. The raw material to make a one-month supply of generic Valtrex® is only 60 cents! The pharmaceutical-quality manufacturing process adds $1.50, which means the total cost to make a bottle of *30* 500 mg generic Valtrex® tablets is only $2.10.

Yet this same bottle retailed in pharmacies for around $200—a government-protected markup of 9,523% (or 95 *times* over the cost of manufacture)!

No other business can get away with charging this much for a product whose patent expired. The only reason this happens is that federal laws provide a virtual monopoly for protecting the drug industry's outlandish profits.

When I called my friend back about the $200/month price, the first thing she said was, "My sister cannot afford that." This means this young girl will suffer frequent herpes outbreaks and is more likely to pass this incurable virus on to others.

For those concerned that this girl may forever be denied her medicine, drug companies have lobbied Congress to create laws whereby taxpayers will foot the bill for many of those who cannot pay the ever-escalating costs of medical insurance.

As we have so often reported, the federal government gives pharmaceutical companies a virtual monopoly over patented and generic drugs. The outlandish profits earned from these drugs are then used to buy lobbyists who persuade Congress to pass legislation that leaves the taxpayer on the hook for paying for these overpriced medicines.

What a racket! Overcharge so much for your product that most consumers cannot afford it, complain to Congress that consumers cannot afford your medicines—and then receive tax dollars to pay your monopolistic prices. We long ago proposed that Congress change the law to permit companies to freely make generics, which would result in the price for generic Valtrex® plummeting from $200 a month to somewhere around $7 (or from $2,400/year to $84/year).

I titled this article "No *Real* Healthcare Cost Crisis" because it reveals how this country is being driven to economic insolvency by corrupt legislation, while pharmaceutical interests enjoy record profits.

MISGUIDED FDA DECISION CAUSES PRICE OF OLD DRUG TO SKYROCKET 5,000%

In July 2009, the FDA officially announced what physicians have long known. An old drug called colchicine can effectively treat acute flares of gouty arthritis.

This drug has been sold as a low-cost generic since the 19th century in the US, and its origins go back 3,000 years to the ancient Greeks.

Since colchicine was around so long, it pre-dated the FDA itself. The FDA wanted this drug tested for safety and efficacy, and offered one company a three-year exclusive if it would conduct a study. In the one-week randomized trial this company conducted, it was discovered that a shortened dosage period produced good symptom management while leading to fewer side effects than longer-term use. Astute physicians may have already figured this out, but it is good that a study was done to confirm the shortened dose advantage. The question is, can we afford it?

Before the study, colchicine was sold by several companies for around nine cents a pill. Once the FDA granted the three-year exclusive, the price shot up 50-fold to an average of $5 per pill.[6]

In 2007, there were 100,000 prescriptions written for colchicine for which Medicare and Medicaid paid about $1 million.[7] Under the new monopoly granted by the FDA (with legislative authority from Congress), taxpayer funded agencies (Medicare and Medicaid) will pay around $50 million for the same drug.[7]

There are more cost-effective ways to have ascertained better dosage for this old drug, such as a one-week trial funded by the National Institutes of Health (NIH). An NIH-funded trial would have cost the government a fraction of the 5,000% *increase* it and private payers will now have to fork over for a non-patented medication that has been used for centuries in this country.

This is just a tiny example of how pharmaceutical company-sponsored legislation and misguided regulatory policies create an artificial healthcare cost crisis. Multiply this across the entire medical sector and you can see why radical reform is needed if an economic crisis it to be averted.

HOW IS THIS AFFECTING YOU?

If you obtain health insurance from your job, it now costs your employer nearly twice as much ($6,700 per employee) than it did in the year 2001.[9] You might have noticed that you now pay a greater portion of the insurance premium through your employer and that your deductibles and co-pays are substantially higher than what they used to be.

Health insurance costs to employers are projected to *double* again over the next ten years. This means that fewer dollars will be available to pay you. It also means that employers are not hiring as many people because of skyrocketing health insurance costs.

Employees fortunate enough to have healthcare insurance in 2010 will pay on average $4,023 in premium subsidies and out-of-pocket expenses.[10] This compares with almost nothing a decade ago. According to the *Wall Street Journal*, "Health Costs Are Crushing Small Businesses," as medical premiums have increased four times faster than the rate of inflation since 2001.[11]

If you pay for your own medical insurance, you've already been stung with skyrocketing premium rate increases, along with higher deductibles, higher co-pays, and refusals to cover certain expenses. Those *without* coverage face astronomical out-of-pocket costs for any serious medical issue.

DRUG MAKERS SHARPLY RAISED PRICES IN 2009

As if prescription drug costs were not already high enough, brand-name pharmaceuticals increased 9.1% in 2009, while biotech drugs rose 11.5%.[8] This follows a pattern of prescription drug price increases that far outpace inflation, even as the cost of the active ingredients plummets (as can be seen in the 60-cent-a-month raw material cost of valacyclovir).

Americans continue to pay the highest prices in the world for their prescription medications, as pharmaceutical company influence in Congress guarantees monopolistic-like protection.

MEDICARE'S DATE WITH INSOLVENCY

According to President Obama, "We will eventually be spending more on Medicare than every other government program combined."[12] That acknowledgment, however, did not stop passage of legislation (The Health Care Reform Act) that provides another Federal disease-care entitlement (and drug company subsidy) for people under age 65. While the public is finally waking up to the colossal $14 trillion official Federal debt, only a few understand that the $24 to $37 trillion unfunded Medicare liability is our real deficit problem. Nothing else comes close to threatening our health and financial well-being.[12]

The year 2008 marked the first time that Medicare posted a deficit, meaning it spent more on disease-care outlays than the taxes it collected. The Federal government tells us that soon the Medicare hospital trust fund will be depleted.[13, 14] But these numbers are based on optimistic projections that are not materializing, such as a 21% cut to doctors that was supposed to occur in 2010 but was canceled by Congress.[13]

An increasing number of doctors are refusing to accept Medicare today because it pays so little. If a cut in physician payments is ever implemented, the Medicare system could collapse because there will not be enough physicians to cover the aging population.

The chart accompanying this article was created in 2007 and reveals the stunning magnitude of the Medicare and Social Security deficits. What's really scary is that this does not factor in the Medicare Prescription Drug Act and The Health Care Reform Act passed by Congress over the past few years that, collectively, will add trillions of additional deficit dollars to this chart.

The Federal government pretends it can raise taxes enough on wealthy individuals to offset the staggering liabilities it has incurred by promising *more* sick-care coverage than what Medicare is already on the hook for. The notion that taxes can be raised on a tiny percentage of the population to pay the gargantuan Medicare liability is a mathematical impossibility and represents the largest Ponzi scheme in the history of mankind.

MEDICARE RIFE WITH FRAUD, WASTE, AND INEPTITUDE

Life Extension® (and other media sources) has reported egregious examples of how Medicare expenditures are squandered. In some cases, crooks set up phony clinics, collect millions from Medicare for services never rendered, and then move on to another location before Medicare figures out it is paying bogus claims.

The real money, however, involves lobbying Congress to force Medicare to grossly overpay for the particular service, device, or pharmaceutical a company happens to sell.

One of the fastest growing areas of the disease-care industry is "home healthcare." It aims to save billions by avoiding costly hospitalizations. Hospitals, of course, learned how to bilk Medicare long ago, and home healthcare providers are no less proficient.

An investigative report by the *Wall Street Journal* uncovered a ridiculous program in which Medicare paid a $2,200 bonus once a company made ten at-home visits to a particular patient.[15] With this kind of incentive, home healthcare companies jumped through hoops to hit the ten-visit mark, even threatening employees with no pay if they failed to figure a way to bill Medicare ten at-home visits for every patient. Remember, for each patient that Medicare paid for ten consecutive visits, an absurd $2,200 taxpayer-funded bonus was kicked back to the home healthcare provider PLUS the cost Medicare had to pay for *each* at-home visit.

Those who successfully lobby Congress receive windfall profits from Medicare, while those who don't are so short-changed that many are dropping out of the system. It's somewhat analogous to the former Soviet Union, where companies favored by the entrenched Communist Party received special status, while those who lacked political connections often could not pay their employees because no money came from Moscow.

One home healthcare company that receives 90% of its revenue payments from Medicare enjoyed revenues of $1.5 billion in 2009, compared to only $88 million in the year 2000. Its stock has gone from less than $1 in 2000 to $60 in 2009.[15]

Clearly, the way to make money in today's economy is to find a way to guarantee that the federal government will pay you inflated prices so you don't have to worry about competing in the free market for consumer dollars.

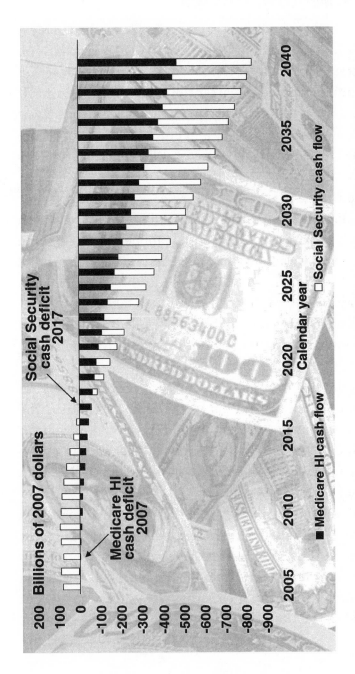

Source: GAO analysis of data from the Office of the Actuary, Social Security Administration and Office of the Actuary, Centers for Medicare and Medcaid Services. Note: Projections based on the intermediate assumptions of the 2007 Trustee's Reports. The CPI is to adjust from current to constant dollares.

A TRIP TO MEXICO WITH MY SON

I try to spend time with my children and wound up in Mexico for a few days last summer, where my 13-year-old son was bitten by an insect. He developed a painful reaction that required immediate attention. Fortunately, in Mexico, you don't need a prescription to buy most drugs. I was able to walk into a pharmacy and purchase a tube of triamcinolone cream at virtually no cost. Within a few hours my son was cured.

In the United States, it is not so easy or affordable. For some ludicrous reason, the FDA mandates that one obtain a doctor's prescription for topically applied triamcinolone cream. If this insect bite had occurred in the US, I would have had to find an urgent care medical facility that was open, pay the doctor over $100, and then take the prescription to a pharmacy and wait for it to be filled. My son would have spent many additional hours in pain and I would have spent a lot more money and time.

If I could not locate an urgent care center, a hospital emergency room visit would be the only alternative. The cost to my insurance company and me would have been over $500 for an ER visit, as opposed to spending only a few dollars for a tube of triamcinolone cream at a Mexican pharmacy with no prescription.

The Mexican pharmacy, by the way, was overwhelmed with American tourists who were behaving like kids in a candy store. The shelves were stocked with just about every popular American prescription drug, but no prescription was required. Prices for most drugs were a fraction of what they cost in the US.

Chase Faloon was bitten by an insect and suffered an acute inflammatory reaction to his entire back on May 27, 2010. Below is the tube of triamcinolone cream I purchased for a few dollars at a Mexican pharmacy (without a prescription) that cured him of the pain, redness, and swelling he suffered. Had this occurred in the United States, this would have been an expensive and time-consuming process.

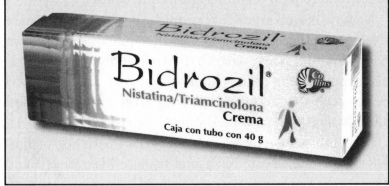

PRESCRIPTION STATUS FOR MANY DRUGS SHOULD BE ABOLISHED

There was a time when the public was so ignorant about medical issues that a doctor's prescription was required for most drugs to be safely and effectively used.

That has changed. An enlightened individual can use the Internet to learn about drugs that lower blood pressure, glucose, and lipids, along with the drug's side effects. At-home blood pressure devices are more effective in monitoring real-world blood pressure than periodic visits to a doctor's office. An enlightened patient can precisely individualize dosing of anti-hypertensive medications to bring their blood pressure to optimal levels (below 115/75 mmHg in most people).

Enlightened individuals, with the help of trained health advisors, can also interpret their own blood test results and choose medications and hormones that can normalize abnormalities that hurried doctors too often overlook. Periodic audits of one's self-prescribing regimen by a physician would be highly recommended.

There are drugs that require close physician supervision and would remain on prescription-only status.

Naysayers who argue that people will take inappropriate doses or the wrong drug ignore the epidemic of adverse reactions that occur when patients blindly follow physicians' prescribing orders. Look at how many prescriptions doctors wrote for Avandia® long after studies showed sharply higher heart attack and stroke risks.[16,17]

If doctors were relieved of having to see patients for simple issues (like elevated LDL and triglycerides), they could focus more time on patients who need intensive, hands-on treatment.

ACCEPTING HARSH REALITIES

Medicare's date with insolvency is a mathematical near-certainty.

There are many reasons for this, but corrupt legislation that precludes a medical free-market from developing, along with bureaucratic over-regulation, ensures that disease-care expenditures will cripple this nation.

As we proposed in detail in the August 2009 issue of *Life Extension Magazine®*, the cost of prescription drugs would plummet if the FDA did not have such stringent approval requirements for generics.

As proposed today, if patients were empowered to make their own decisions on personal health issues, medical costs would plunge as wasteful visits to doctors' offices could be reduced.

I suspect most of you reading this recognize that there comes a point where the words "we cannot afford it" become a harsh reality. Whether one agrees with the solutions suggested in this editorial or not, the simple fact is that Medicare, private insurance, and the private sector cannot afford the costs of today's broken sick-care system.

For the edification of new members, please know that we at Life Extension® have been sounding the alarm bells about the catastrophic consequences of artificially inflated disease-care costs for the past four decades.

The Federal government has responded by launching relentless criminal investigations against me (and others) at the behest of pharmaceutical interests, who don't want you to know that Americans have been forced to pay $200 for a bottle of valacyclovir (Valtrex®) that costs only $2.10 to make!

Please note that generic drug prices fluctuate widely. When more manufacturers obtain FDA approval, prices sometimes drop. When manufacturers cease making certain generics, prices can sharply increase. In January 2011, the Life Extension® Pharmacy® was able to offer 30 500 mg tablets of valacyclovir for $103, though this price is subject to being increased at any time. When I called a local Walgreens the very same day, they quoted $199.99 for the same amount of valacyclovir.

Note: From an efficacy standpoint, valacyclovir provides relatively mediocre results in those suffering acute herpes or shingles outbreaks.

References

1. Faloon W. How much more FDA abuse can Americans tolerate? *Life Extension Magazine®*. 2010 Mar;16(3):12–3.
2. Faloon W. Startling findings about vitamin D levels in Life Extension® members. *Life Extension Magazine®*. 2010 Jan;16(1):7–14.

3. Faloon W. Why American healthcare is headed for collapse. *Life Extension Magazine®*. 2009 Sep;15(9):7–12.

4. Available at: http://www.cdc.gov/std/herpes/stdfact-herpes. htm#common. Accessed July 7, 2010.

5. Lebrun-Vignes B, Bouzamondo A, Dupuy A, Guillaume JC, Lechat P, Chosidow O. A meta-analysis to assess the efficacy of oral antiviral treatment to prevent genital herpes outbreaks. *J Am Acad Dermatol*. 2007 Aug;57(2):238–46.

6. Kesselheim AS, Solomon DH. Incentives for drug development—the curious case of colchicine. *N Engl J Med*. 2010 Jun 3;362(22):2045–7.

7. Available at: http://www.urlpharma.com/url_unapproved_drug_NEJM.aspx. Accessed July, 2010.

8. Available at:http://online.wsj.com/article/SB100014240527 4870375750457519443232875278.html. Accessed November 19, 2010.

9. Available at: http://www.commonwealthfund.org/usr_doc/ Collins_whitheremployer-basedhltins_1059.pdf. Accessed November 24, 2010.

10. Available at: http://online.wsj.com/article/SB100014240527 48703790404574471290259603238.html. Accessed November 24, 2010.

11. Available at: http://online.wsj.com/article/SB100014240527 48703298004574455321821703370.html. Accessed November 24, 2010.

12. Available at: http://online.wsj.com/article/SB100014240529 70203440104574404893691325078.html. Accessed November 24, 2010.

13. Available at:http://online.wsj.com/article/SB124212734686110365. html. Accessed November 24, 2010.

14. Available at: http://online.wsj.com/article/SB100014240529 70204884404574362543878647858.html. Accessed November 24, 2010.

15. Available at: http://online.wsj.com/article/SB100014240527 48703625304575116040870004462.html. Accessed December 2, 2010.

16. Available at: http://diabetes.webmd.com/news/20100628/ new-study-avandia-riskier-than-actos. Accessed November 24, 2010.

17. Available at: http://prescriptions.blogs.nytimes.com/2010/07/14/ blogging-the-f-d-a-panel-on-avandia/. Accessed November 24, 2010.

2010

FDA Delay of One Drug Causes 82,000 Lost Life-Years

Reviewed and critiqued by STEPHEN B. STRUM, MD,
FACP, Medical Oncologist specializing in
prostate cancer since 1983

I N 2004, I WROTE AN ARTICLE describing how Americans die needlessly because of the FDA's delay in approving life-saving drugs.[1]

One example of a delayed therapy I cited was Provenge®, which in the year 2002 had demonstrated improved survival in prostate cancer patients.[2]

In 2007, Dr. Stephen Strum and I co-authored an article showing how enormous numbers of lives could be spared if scientists were liberated from oppressive FDA over-regulation. We described several cancer drugs that should have been approved including Provenge®, which by the year 2007 had extended survival in several clinical studies.[3]

In 2010, the FDA finally approved Provenge®.[4] This was after still another FDA-mandated clinical trial documented the efficacy of this therapy.

As you're about to read, the FDA's eight-year delay in approving Provenge® has resulted in a horrific number of prostate cancer victims prematurely dying!

HOW EFFECTIVE IS PROVENGE®?

Once the FDA finally approved Provenge® in April 2010, the news media hailed it as a miracle new cancer therapy. What the media failed to convey was the fact that Provenge® was not new. It had been discovered almost a decade earlier. Despite the impressive study results you are about to read, the FDA denied it for eight long years.

In an analysis from the first study in 2002, Provenge®-treated men with a less aggressive prostate cancer (Gleason score 7 or less) were eight times *more* likely to live six months without disease progression compared to placebo.[2]

After 30 months, these same patients receiving Provenge® were 3.7 times more likely to be alive. This translates into 53% of the Provenge® group surviving compared to only 14% of the placebo group. The Provenge® group also remained pain-free twice as long on average as the placebo group.[2,3]

The FDA refused to recognize these findings and ordered the company to conduct more clinical studies. We at Life Extension® were livid at the time over the FDA's decision to deny prostate cancer patients access to this therapy.

Fast forward to 2005, and the results of a new clinical study showed that three times as many advanced prostate cancer patients who received Provenge® were alive compared to patients receiving a placebo.[5,6]

This study evaluated 127 patients with prostate cancer that did not respond to androgen-deprivation therapy. Cancer experts consider this patient subset to have a dismal prognosis, with most dying of the disease within a few years. In this Provenge® study, 34% of the patients receiving Provenge® were still alive after three years compared to only 11% of men who were randomly assigned a placebo.[5] The FDA again refused to approve Provenge®, even with this kind of data in hand.

In the most recent study on advanced prostate cancer patients, Provenge® prolonged median survival by 4.5 months and produced a greater than threefold increase in survival at 36 months compared to placebo.[7]

As I'll explain later, any improvement in survival in advanced cancer cases is viewed favorably, as these patients have already failed grueling conventional therapies. We postulate that if used earlier in the disease process and in combination with other non-toxic therapies, Provenge® will be far more effective.

Based on this latest study and in conjunction with the other prior favorable studies, the FDA finally approved Provenge®—eight years later than it should have!

HOW MANY LIFE-YEARS LOST BECAUSE OF FDA'S DELAY?

Prostate cancer killed 27,360 American men in 2009.[8] This is down from prior years where it used to kill around 30,000 Americans. Earlier diagnosis is one reason for this decline. Far fewer men are diagnosed with advanced prostate cancer with bone metastases today because of PSA testing.

In determining how many human life-years have been lost because of the FDA's delay in approving Provenge®, we would come up with very high numbers if we only used data from the most favorable studies.

Instead, we choose to use the least favorable data that looked only at median survival improvement in those with advanced stage prostate cancer who were no longer responding to conventional therapy.

We took the low number of 27,360 men who died of prostate cancer in 2009 and multiplied it times the 4.5 months of improved survival demonstrated in the latest study. The total number of human life-years lost *each year* the FDA delayed approving Provenge® comes out to 10,260.

Multiply the eight years the FDA delayed approving Provenge®, and the total number of lost life-years is a startling 82,080. To state this statistic differently, 82,080 lost life-years translates to 1,066 entire lives lost. This calculation is based on taking the 82,080 lost life-years divided by average male life expectancy of 77 years.

The federal government refuses to consider Life Extension's longstanding recommendation of making FDA approval voluntary, as opposed to the compulsory process it is today.

If prostate cancer victims had access to Provenge® when it first demonstrated efficacy in 2002, 82,000 human life-years could have been spared.

PROVENGE® IS JUST ONE OF MANY DELAYED DRUGS

The cover story of the September 2007 issue of *Life Extension Magazine®* was titled "Life-saving Cancer Drugs Rejected by the FDA." In that issue, we meticulously described several anti-cancer drugs (including Provenge®) the FDA had not yet approved. All of these drugs had substantial scientific evidence indicating efficacy. We argued that since terminal cancer patients had no other options, they should be allowed access to these therapies.

In the case of Provenge®, an FDA advisory panel recommended it be approved in the year 2007.[9,10] FDA bureaucrats, however, ignored scientists on this advisory panel and mandated that more studies be done.

FDA DELAY MAKES PROVENGE® COST-PROHIBITIVE

Had Provenge® been made available in 2002, like it could have been, it might be available at a more reasonable price today. The FDA's insistence on multiple redundant clinical studies will result in the therapy costing $93,000 per patient.

Medicare recently stated they will pay for Provenge®, though some private insurance companies may balk. Either way, consumers will pay for the FDA's delay in the form of higher medical insurance premiums, higher taxes, and/or having to pay for the drug out of pocket.

As we have stated many times, a key factor in today's healthcare financial crisis is that medical progress and efficiency are obstructed by bureaucratic delays leading to hyper-inflated costs.

WE WERE NOT THE ONLY ONES SCREAMING FOR PROVENGE® TO BE APPROVED

The FDA was put under enormous pressure to approve Provenge® ever since the first successful clinical study came out in the year 2002. After a second study showed even greater efficacy, prostate cancer support groups, scientific organizations, and even mainstream publications demanded that the FDA grant terminal patients the right to try this therapy.

The January 26, 2004 issue of the *Wall Street Journal* featured an editorial stating:

> We know that it works, and we know why it works. In any rational regulatory environment, that would be reason to speed Provenge® to market.[11]

By 2007, there was a revolt underway against the FDA for continuing to reject Provenge®, including threats by members of Congress to conduct a full-scale investigation and lawsuits filed by patient support groups. FDA bureau-crats, however, steadfastly refused to budge (until April 29, 2010).[12]

Even though Provenge® therapy is now officially approved, it will only be available to treat about 2,000 patients over the next year.[13] That's because it requires specialized laboratories to be established throughout the United States to take each cancer patient's blood and create an individualized vaccine. The problem is that more than 27,000 men will die of prostate cancer over the next twelve months, meaning that fewer than 8% of these fellow human beings will have access to Provenge® before they die.

HOW THE FDA STIFLES NEW CANCER DRUG DEVELOPMENT

When an experimental therapy prolongs life by only a few months in advanced cancer cases, the public often assumes the treatment is of little value.

The reason new cancer therapies often show mediocre results in clinical studies is that the FDA mandates that these new drugs only be tested in advanced-stage patients who have failed currently approved therapies. This creates a major obstacle because therapies that might cure cancer (or induce durable remissions) if used in earlier stages may be ineffective in advanced stages of the disease.

Once the drug is approved, however, it can be used (off-label) sometimes more effectively in treating earlier-stage disease patients. It can also be used in combination with other therapies to yield better survival results, something that is usually not allowed in clinical trial designs the FDA tightly controls.

The reason that it is so difficult to kill advanced-stage, treatment-resistant cancers is that they have mutated and acquired multiple survival mechanisms. These advanced-stage cancer cells are thus extremely difficult to eradicate with any therapy.

Now that Provenge® has been approved by the FDA, innovative oncologists can prescribe it for early-stage prostate cancer patients whose cancers have not developed a resistance to androgen deprivation therapy. These earlier-stage patients may respond better than the advanced hormone refractory cases on which the drug was tested in the clinical trials.

When one understands the many roadblocks the FDA erects against promising cancer treatments, it becomes clear why more effective therapies have not been discovered to eradicate this insidious disease.

In an ideal setting, Provenge® would have been made available to those who wished to "opt-out" of the FDA's regulatory stranglehold, and we would have learned long ago how effective Provenge® therapy was against a wide range of prostate cancers.

At this point, we don't even know how effective Provenge® will be outside the clinical study setting. Not all drugs shown effective in tightly controlled studies are as efficacious in the real world. Getting drugs out faster will enable those dealing with real-world cancer patients to ascertain safety and efficacy.

FDA INTERFERENCE WORSE THAN WHAT MOST EXPERTS THINK

For the past 30 years, Life Extension® has identified effective medications that languished too long in the FDA's archaic approval process.

When lifesaving new drugs are delayed, the inevitable consequence is needless human suffering and death. An equally insidious problem is the chilling effect that bureau-cratic roadblocks have on the development of better drugs that might cure the disease.

Just imagine the difficulty of raising the tens of millions of dollars needed to get a new cancer drug into the approval pipeline when prospective investors see the FDA delay a drug with documented efficacy for eight years, as was done with Provenge®.

Another problem with the FDA's unpredictable approval pattern is the outrageous cost of cancer drugs that do make it to market. Insurance companies do not always pay for these new drugs, thus forcing desperate cancer victims to pay out-of-pocket for new drugs that can exceed $12,000 per month. The media has reported on heart-wrenching stories of cancer patients who choose to die rather than condemn their families to bankruptcy in order to pay these costs.

It's easy to point fingers at drug companies for charging such extortionist prices, but the harsh reality is that getting these medications approved by the FDA is so costly and risky that the high prices can arguably be justified by the inefficient drug approval process that now exists.

WHY DRUGS LIKE PROVENGE® TAKE SO LONG TO APPROVE

The fundamental problem with today's byzantine drug approval process is bureaucratic inefficiency and corruption.

What the public does not understand is that when a new therapy like Provenge® is being considered for approval, companies selling older (less effective) drugs have a tremendous incentive to block the better medicine. It can be quite cost-effective to persuade the FDA to erect barriers against newer therapies that compete with highly profitable existing drugs.

Allegations ran rampant that the FDA delayed Provenge® because large pharmaceutical companies did not want to lose revenue from toxic chemotherapy drugs that advanced prostate cancer patients were forced to use in lieu of Provenge®.

Bureaucratic ineptitude has been highlighted by the failures of the Securities and Exchange Commission (SEC) to prevent widespread financial fraud.[14] As you may know, even when outsiders conducted meticulous investigations and handed cases like that of Ponzi schemer Bernie Madoff to the SEC on a silver platter, the SEC did nothing to stop Madoff from defrauding more victims.

When complaints are made about FDA drug delays, a knee-jerk response from some in Congress is, "we need to give the FDA more money." It is regrettable that politicians can't see past the simple fact that providing more money and power to incompetent and corrupt agencies results in more incompetence and corruption.

THIS IS NO LONGER A DEBATABLE ISSUE

Provenge® is by no means the first drug Life Extension® recommended years or decades before the FDA permitted it to be sold to Americans. For example, we fought for nearly two decades to force the FDA to approve ribavirin as an adjuvant treatment for hepatitis C, and low-dose aspirin for heart attack prevention. In both cases, we faced criminal investigations by FDA agents who felt it more productive to put us in jail rather than approve these lifesaving therapies.

Sadly, most of the drugs Life Extension® has identified as having probable efficacy are never allowed on the American market because the sponsor company runs out of money jumping over the FDA's impossibly high regulatory hurdles.

POTENTIAL OF PROVENGE® RECOGNIZED
LONG BEFORE FDA APPROVAL

In 2002, Stephen Strum, MD and Donna Pogliano, the significant other of a man with prostate cancer, published a book entitled *The Primer on Prostate Cancer* (Life Extension® Media, 2002). Within that outstanding guide to prostate cancer diagnosis and management, a section was devoted to "Treatments on the Horizon." The very first treatment discussed in detail was Provenge®.

We now know that if Americans had the freedom to try Provenge® as early as the year 2002, countless numbers of premature deaths could have been prevented. (*The Primer on Prostate Cancer* is still in print and available from Life Extension®.)

The FDA now says (in 2010) that Provenge® is effective in prolonging survival in men with advanced prostate cancer. That means the drug was also effective in the year 2002, when the FDA first suppressed it.

With Provenge® (and many other drugs), there is nothing more to debate. The FDA's delay of this one drug caused the equivalent loss of over 1,000 entire lives. This is the same as terrorists killing 1,000 newborn babies, yet no one in the media even suggested that the FDA was tardy in approving Provenge®. Americans can no longer tolerate this ongoing atrocity, either from a financial or morality standpoint.

WHAT YOU CAN DO TO STOP
NEEDLESS CANCER DEATHS

Scientists have identified novel ways of treating cancer, but too little of this new technology is being used in clinical practice. When new discoveries are made, drug companies spend years seeking a patent, and then more years carrying the drug through the cumbersome bureaucratic approval process. A major reason so many cancer patients die today is an antiquated regulatory system that causes effective therapies to be delayed (or suppressed altogether).

This system must be changed if the 1,500 American cancer patients who would perish each day are to have a realistic chance of being saved.

Our longstanding proposal has been to change the law so that anyone can opt out of the FDA's umbrella of "protection." This approach will allow companies to sell drugs that have demonstrated safety and a reasonable likelihood of effectiveness, which are clearly labeled "Not Approved by the FDA." Patients who wish can still use only FDA-approved drugs, while those willing to take a risk, in consultation with their doctors, will be allowed to try drugs shown to be safe that are still not approved.

We believe that this initiative will result in a renaissance in the practice of medicine similar to the computer technology revolution of the past three decades. In the liberated environment we propose, many lethal diseases will succumb to cures that are less expensive than is presently the case. And greater competition will help eliminate the healthcare cost crisis that exists today.

Today's broken system results in terminally ill people learning of scientific discoveries that might well cure their disease, but sadly hearing their newscaster say the therapy is years away from FDA approval. We think that seriously ill people, in consultation with their doctors, should be able to make up their own minds about what drugs they are willing to try.

LEGISLATION THAT WOULD HAVE MADE LIFESAVING THERAPIES AVAILABLE SOONER

For the past three decades, Life Extension® has sought to expose an insidious drug approval process that causes human beings to die, even though effective therapies to treat their diseases already exist.

THE ABIGAIL ALLIANCE: A RELENTLESS CAMPAIGN TO REFORM THE FDA

The Compassionate Access Act of 2010 was introduced into Congress based on the relentless efforts of an organization called The Abigail Alliance.

This non-profit organization was founded based on the heart-wrenching events surrounding a young girl (Abigail Burroughs) who was denied access to what the FDA now admits is an effective cancer drug.

Abigail Burroughs was diagnosed at age 19 with a squamous cell carcinoma that had invaded her neck and lungs. Abigail was an honor student and high school athlete, a confident yet humble person who was wise beyond her years. And she was compassionate, devoting much of her young life to charity work, making beds at homeless shelters and creating a free tutoring program for 50 families who couldn't afford tutors. Abigail had a great love of life and a deep respect for all beings.

Not long after her diagnosis, the Burroughs family learned of an investigational cancer drug that showed good response in early trials. Abigail's prominent oncologist at Johns Hopkins Hospital believed the drug had a significant chance of saving her life. But every effort on the part of her family, physician, and supporters to procure the drug for Abigail failed. She was ineligible for a clinical trial and the drug company couldn't provide it for her for compassionate use. The FDA was unmoved by her life-and-death situation.

In November 2000, Abigail was recovering from a round of chemotherapy and radiation treatment when she said to her father, "Dad, if I make it, I'd like you and I to devote our lives to helping people with cancer and other illnesses where there's an unmet need." After seven months of battling to acquire the experimental drug for Abigail, she died, her young life tragically cut short by an indifferent system that has cost an untold number of lives. The drug was later approved by the FDA as being effective against her type of cancer.

Hours after she died, through his tremendous grief, her father Frank Burroughs realized that the inability of seriously ill patients to obtain effective drugs still under study was a critical unmet need. His daughter had wanted to help not only herself, but others like her, and Burroughs knew then that he had to continue fighting the system.

Burroughs explained, "Hundreds of thousands of Americans die every year awaiting drug approval, a catastrophe of immense proportions. I said to myself, 'Why should I quit now? There are other people out there who are just as precious as Abigail.' She had planted the seed of an idea. She was the embodiment of the unmet need. But we certainly weren't the only ones."

To learn more about the Abigail Alliance, log on to: http://www.abigail-alliance.org/.

The Compassionate Access Act of 2010 (H.R. 4732) did not pass in the 111th Congress, but its supporters plan to reintroduce it.

The FDA is able to suppress innovative therapies because the public has failed to demand that our elected officials rein in the FDA's arbitrary authority. The first step in changing today's outmoded system is to communicate the urgent need for change to Congress.

A bill titled the Compassionate Access Act of 2010 (H.R. 4732) was introduced into the House of Representatives in 2010.[16] This bill would have amended the Food, Drug, and Cosmetic Act to create a new conditional approval system for drugs, biological products, and devices for seriously ill patients.

While this bill would not have enabled patients to "opt-out" of the FDA's regulatory stranglehold, it was an important first step that will demonstrate that human lives can be spared if earlier access to experimental therapies is permitted.

We expect this bill will be reintroduced and will encourage Life Extension® supporters to support it, as passage of this legislation will enable cancer patients (and others with serious diseases) to obtain therapies far enough along in the clinical trials process to be deemed safe, but not yet approved by the FDA.

We at Life Extension® have long contended that any person with a serious illness should have the individual right to choose therapies that have not yet received official FDA approval.

References

1. Faloon W. Are you afraid of terrorists? *Life Extension Magazine®*. 2004 Jun;10(6):9–15.
2. Available at: http://findarticles.com/p/articles/mi_m0EIN/is_2002_Dec_11/ai_95190631/. Accessed June 29, 2010.
3. Faloon W, Strum S. FDA rejects promising prostate cancer drug. *Life Extension Magazine®*. 2007 Sept;13(9):7–12.
4. Available at: http://www.fda.gov/News Events/Newsroom/PressAnnouncements/ucm210174.htm. Accessed August 4, 2010.
5. Small EJ, Schellhammer PF, Higano CS, et al. Placebo-controlled phase III trialof immunologic therapy with sipuleucel-T (APC8015) in patients with metastatic, asymptomatic hormone refractory prostate cancer. J Clin Oncol. 2006 Jul 1;24(19):3089–94.
6. Available at: http://www.psa-rising.com/med/immun/provenge-05.htm. Accessed August 5, 2010.
7. Higano CS, Schellhammer PF, Small EJ, et al. Integrated data from 2 randomized, double-blind, placebo-controlled, phase 3 trials of active cellular immunotherapy with sipuleucel-T in advanced prostate cancer. *Cancer*. 2009 Aug 15;115(16):3670–9.
8. Available at: http://www.medicinenet.com/script/main/art.asp?articlekey=100730. Accessed August 5, 2010.

9. Available at: http://www.cnn.com/2010/HEALTH/04/27/provenge.prostate.cancer.fda/index.html. Accessed August 5, 2010.

10. Available at:http://www.fda.gov/NewsEvents/Newsroom/PressAnnouncements/ucm210174.htm. Accessed August 5, 2010.

11. New cancer drugs. *Wall Street Journal*. January 26, 2004.

12. Available at: http://caretolive.com/2008-01-20/fda-under-pressure-from-congress-to-explain-provenge-delay/. Accessed June 29, 2010.

13. Available at: http://www.medscape.com/viewarticle/721160. Accessed July 1, 2010.

14. Available at: http://www.dailyfinance.com/story/media/how-madoff-got-away-with-it-sec-report-phone-transcript-reveal/19156812/. Accessed July 1, 2010

15. Available at: http://www.cnn.com/2010/POLITICS/04/23/sec.porn/index.html. Accessed July 2, 2010.

16. Available at: http://www.abigail-alliance.org/S_3046_ACCESS_Act.pdf. Accessed July 2, 2010.

Deadly FDA Neglect

YOU MIGHT BE SURPRISED to learn that the leading cause of acute liver failure in the United States is neither alcohol abuse, nor viral hepatitis.

The number one reason Americans suffer acute liver failure is a drug the FDA has allowed to be sold for decades after its lethal toxicities were known.[1]

This drug is available over-the-counter and in prescription combinations. In many cases, those ingesting this toxic drug (under various brand names) don't even know they are taking it.

The FDA has bent over backwards to protect billions of dollars of profits earned annually by pharmaceutical companies who sell this deadly drug.

As the body count mounted in 2009, the FDA was forced to mandate a lower dosage and remove it from prescription combinations that were particularly lethal.[2]

The FDA's feeble actions to appease critics are too little and far too late. The reduced dose will spare some lives, but this toxic drug will still inflict a considerable death toll. The fact that this carnage has gone on for decades confirms the FDA's blatant failure to protect the public.

WHAT CALLED MY ATTENTION TO THIS DRUG-INDUCED BLOODBATH?

Back in the early 1980s, I was having one of my all-night brainstorming sessions with scientists who routinely think "outside the box" when it comes to medical issues. One of these scientists enlightened me as to the mechanism by which the pain reliever acetaminophen causes liver damage.

When acetaminophen is ingested, a rapid depletion of glutathione in the liver occurs.[3,4] The result of glutathione depletion is free-radical destruction of liver cells.[5–9] The scientists I spoke with suggested that Life Extension® make a combination product of acetaminophen and N-acetyl cysteine (a glutathione-enhancing amino acid). According to these scientists, this would probably eliminate virtually all acetaminophen-related acute deaths.[10–14]

Since acetaminophen and N-acetyl cysteine are both sold over-the-counter, you might think that making a "safer" acetaminophen formula would not be difficult.

There is one problem. The FDA prohibits combining existing drugs and dietary supplements unless a New Drug Application is filed, tens of millions of dollars of clinical studies are performed, and the FDA agrees to allow the combination to be sold. The whole process can cost upwards of $100 million and take a decade to complete.

So, by bureaucratic edict, a safer form of acetaminophen never made it to market.

FDA THROWS US IN JAIL!

In the late 1980s, the FDA began raiding our facilities for the purposes of gathering evidence to put my colleagues and me in jail. According to the FDA, our products were not approved by the agency and were therefore inherently unsafe.

We fought back by showing that not only were the products we recommended safe and effective, but that many of the drugs the FDA claimed to be safe were really poisons!

We were indicted in the early 1990s under charges that our product recommendations violated the FDA's coveted regulatory structure, which included having approved labeling so consumers and their doctors could safely use these products.

MY WEEKLY RADIO SHOW

In response to those who believed the FDA's fabricated attacks against us, I set up my own radio show on one of the largest stations in South Florida.

Almost every week I would identify a drug the FDA approved as "safe" and reveal just how dangerous it really was. I would then discuss ways to make these drugs safer, such as taking coenzyme Q10 if a statin cholesterol-lowering drug were needed. It was known way back then that statin drugs interfere with CoQ10 synthesis in the body.[15] By taking supplemental CoQ10, those taking statin drugs could replenish their bodies with this life-sustaining nutrient that is depleted by statins and aging.

In recalling my conversations with forward-thinking scientists in the early 1980s, I researched acetaminophen and was astounded by the multiple toxic effects this drug inflicts on the liver,[16-20] kidney,[21-26] and other organs.[27-29]

When I went to the pharmacy to check out the labeling, there were no warnings required by the FDA to indicate this drug's lethal side effects.

So here I was facing decades in prison for recommending products that did not have FDA-approved labeling, yet the FDA did not require labeling for one of the most dangerous drugs on the market to warn consumers about its lethal effects.

These egregious disparities were not lost on prosecutors, who eventually dismissed the FDA's flawed indictments against us.

JUST HOW DANGEROUS IS ACETAMINOPHEN?

Each year, acetaminophen poisoning results in 100,000 calls to poison control centers, 56,000 emergency room visits, 26,000 hospitalizations, and more than 450 deaths from liver failure.[30]

Acetaminophen's deadly effects extend beyond the liver. Regular users of acetaminophen may double their risk of kidney cancer, a disease that kills 12,000 Americans each year.[25, 26, 31-33] The incidence of kidney cancer in the US has risen 126% since the 1950s,[34] a jump that may be tied to the growing use of drugs containing acetaminophen and its metabolites.

Because acetaminophen generates damaging free radicals throughout the body, it may very well increase the risk of many age-related diseases. In fact, scientists can consistently induce cataracts in the eyes of laboratory animals by giving them acetaminophen.[35] They consider acetaminophen a "cataractogenic agent." Interestingly, if antioxidants are provided to the animals, the cataract-inducing effects[36-40] of acetaminophen are often completely neutralized.[41, 42]

Just imagine how the FDA would respond if a dietary supplement caused even a few of these adverse reactions. The FDA would immediately shut down the company and probably pursue criminal charges against the owners. Not so with acetaminophen. Since it is "approved" by the FDA, little has been done until now to restrict consumer access to it.

FDA SCIENTIFIC ADVISORY PANEL
RECOGNIZES RISKS

In 2009, an outside advisory panel recommended that the FDA ban narcotics containing acetaminophen.[43] The panel also recommended that the amount of acetaminophen contained in OTC products be reduced.

The FDA's response to its own Scientific Advisory Panel was to implement some changes to protect Americans against the liver damage inflicted by over-the-counter and prescription acetaminophen drugs.[44, 45] No mention was made about combining acetaminophen with N-acetyl cysteine to protect against glutathione depletion and subsequent free radical-induced liver damage. There was also no mention about the other health problems (like kidney failure and kidney cancer) potentially caused by acetaminophen.

The most popular acetaminophen-containing drug is Tylenol®, and its makers wasted no time in running full-page ads proclaiming that Tylenol® remains the "safest" pain-relieving drug on the market. There appears to be no limit to how low pharmaceutical companies will sink to protect their immoral profits. To imply that acetaminophen is "safe" is a scientific contradiction.

ACETAMINOPHEN AND THE FDA:
A SORDID HISTORY

The 2009 announcement about acetaminophen's deadly effects is not the first time an independent group of doctors recommended the FDA do something about this drug.

In 2002, another independent advisory committee commissioned by the FDA urged that warnings be put on the labels of acetaminophen drugs.[46,47] The FDA said no to its own scientific advisors. Instead, the FDA budgeted a mere twenty thousand dollars[29, 30] to develop material that it hoped would be run in magazines and distributed by pharmacy chains for free![48] This is the bureaucratic equivalent of doing nothing.

By 2004, the FDA capitulated to scientific pressure and mandated a minimal warning be placed on acetaminophen labels, which did nothing to stop the slaughter caused by this deadly drug.[49]

FDA SHOULD HAVE KNOWN ABOUT KIDNEY TOXICITY

The painkiller drug phenacetin was taken off the market long ago because of its severe kidney toxicity and its association with an increased risk of bladder cancer.[50-54] Acetaminophen is the major metabolite of this banned drug, meaning that phenacetin's destructive properties may have been caused by its breakdown to acetaminophen in the body. So while phenacetin was withdrawn because too many peoples' kidneys were shutting down, the FDA had no problem letting its major metabolite (acetaminophen) be freely marketed without any consumer warning whatsoever.

If acetaminophen is responsible for even a small percentage of the overall annual kidney cancer cases, the FDA's failure to restrict this one drug may have killed tens of thousands of Americans from this one disease alone!

As history has taught us, when a highly profitable drug turns out to be a lethal killer, the FDA's first response is to safeguard pharmaceutical economic interests. Consumer protection is a secondary issue.

IT IS "IMPOSSIBLE" FOR THE FDA TO PROTECT THE PUBLIC

Life Extension® warned about the lethal dangers of acetaminophen-containing drugs almost 20 years ago. The FDA carefully listened to each one of my radio shows hoping to identify new criminal charges they could bring against me, but did nothing to alert the public about acetaminophen's deadly side effects. Even when national news broadcasts reported on real-life victims who died from acetaminophen, the agency responsible for protecting Americans against unsafe drugs stood still. Why was that?

As most of you know, pharmaceutical interests exert tremendous control over the FDA. Employees of the FDA are offered lucrative pharmaceutical jobs upon retirement and are heavily lobbied by drug companies while working at the agency.

Members of Congress charged with overseeing the FDA are also inundated by pharmaceutical industry lobbyists and campaign contributions. When the safety of a drug as popular as acetaminophen is challenged, you can be certain pharmaceutical companies will pull out all the stops to make sure the government does not ban it.

Even when the FDA proposes stricter labeling on drugs like acetaminophen, pharmaceutical lobbyists besiege the FDA and Congress to make these warnings so benign that the public largely ignores them.

The degree of political influence involved in FDA decision-making results in it being impossible for the agency to use scientific evidence to protect Americans against unsafe drugs.

As I described earlier in this article, those not beholden to the pharmaceutical cartel learned of acetaminophen's lethal effects decades ago—and even came up with preventive antidotes (such as N-acetyl cysteine). Yet to this day, acetaminophen continues to poison huge segments of the American public who still are unaware of how toxic this drug really is.

ALL PAIN-SUPPRESSING MEDICATIONS ARE TOXIC

To relieve chronic pain, toxic doses of all approved analgesics are often required. That argument has been used by acetaminophen makers to state that if patients have to switch to other FDA-approved drugs (such as ibuprofen or Celebrex®), then users will die from other causes, such as stomach bleeding and heart attacks.

We don't disagree that all FDA-approved pain relievers are dangerous and only minimally effective. We question why conventional doctors liberally prescribe toxic analgesics without seeking to alleviate the underlying cause of the pain.

In some cases, chiropractic care can result in functional and symptom relief of chronic pain. Certain dietary supplements such as gamma-linolenic acid (from borage oil),[55] high-dose fish oil,[56, 57] MSM (methylsulphonylmethane),[58, 59] and Korean Angelica extract[60,61] have demonstrated remarkable pain- relieving effects in peer-reviewed published scientific studies.

In 2009, we introduced an infrared heating pad that delivers a steady stream of soothing warmth deep into the tissues. We sold ten times more of these infrared pads than we expected, and have received remarkable testimonials back from users. The number of these infrared pads we shipped out indicates how many people suffer from chronic pain. Unfortunately, the FDA decided to ban the importation of this product until the company completes lengthy and burdensome registration requirements, so many of those suffering chronic pain will have no choice but to resort to toxic drugs the FDA allows to be freely sold. We will let you know if and when these infrared heating pads ever become available.

FREE MARKET MORE EFFECTIVE THAN FDA

For more than a century, consumers have been misled into believing the FDA protected them against dangerous drugs. The harsh reality is that the FDA functions to protect the economic interests of the pharmaceutical establishment, while trampling on the rights of Americans to access safer and more effective natural therapies.

**UPDATE: THE FDA FINALLY ACTS ...
BUT TOO LITTLE, TOO LATE**

It has taken almost twenty years from our initial warning, but in January 2011 the FDA finally announced that it will limit the amount of acetaminophen allowed in prescription painkillers such as Vicodin® and Percocet®. The FDA is also asking makers of acetaminophen to add the strongest possible warning—a black box—to their labels about the possibility of severe liver damage.

Strangely, this dose reduction and black box warning will not apply to over-the-counter acetaminophen products like Tylenol® and hundreds of cold, flu, and other pain relievers sold to unsuspecting consumers with no physician supervision.

The mandates on prescription acetaminophen drugs will be phased in over three years, meaning the FDA is in no hurry to protect Americans from prescription acetaminophen's deadly effects.

These new FDA mandates are less stringent than what its own scientific advisory committee recommended, which wanted prescription drugs like Vicodin® and Percocet® to be banned altogether.

All of this provides another piece of irrefutable evidence that the FDA functions to protect the outrageous profits of pharmaceutical companies like Johnson and Johnson instead of the lives of innocent Americans.

References

1. Bromer MQ, Black M. Acetaminophen hepatotoxicity. *Clin Liver Dis.* 2003 May;7(2):351–67.

2. Available at: http://www.time.com/time/health/article/0,8599,1908042,00.html. Accessed July 16, 2009.

3. Wu J, Danielsson A, Zern MA. Toxicity of hepatotoxins: new insights into mechanisms and therapy. *Expert Opin Investig Drugs.* 1999 May;8(5):585–607.

4. Richie JP Jr, Lang CA, Chen TS. Acetaminophen-induced depletion of glutathione and cysteine in the aging mouse kidney. *Biochem Pharmacol.* 1992 Jul 7;44(1):129–35.

5. DeLeve LD, Kaplowitz N. Glutathione metabolism and its role in hepatotoxicity. *Pharmacol Ther.* 1991 Dec;52(3):287–305.

6. Larson AM, Polson J, Fontana RJ, et al. Acetaminophen-induced acute liver failure: results of a United States multicenter, prospective study. *Hepatology.* 2005; 42(6):1364–72.

7. Uhlig S, Wendel A. Glutathione enhancement in various mouse organs and protection by glutathione isopropyl ester against liver injury. *Biochem Pharmacol.* 1990 Jun 15;39(12):1877–81.

8. Loguercio C, Del Vecchio Blanco C, Coltorti M, Nardi G. Alteration of erythrocyte glutathione, cysteine and glutathione synthetase in alcoholic and non-alcoholic cirrhosis. *Scand J Clin Lab Invest.* 1992 May;52(3):207–13.

9. Shigesawa T, Sato C, Marumo F. Significance of plasma glutathione determination in patients with alcoholic and non-alcoholic liver disease. *J Gastroenterol Hepatol.* 1992 Jan-Feb;7(1):7–11.

10. Atkuri KR, Mantovani JJ, Herzenberg LA, Herzenberg LA. N-Acetylcysteine—a safe antidote for cysteine/glutathione deficiency. *Curr Opin Pharmacol.* 2007 Aug;7(4):355–9.

11. Millea PJ. N-acetylcysteine: multiple clinical applications. *Am Fam Physician.* 2009 Aug 1;80(3):265–9.

12. Tsai CL, Chang WT, Weng TI, Fang CC, Walson PD. A patient-tailored N-acetylcysteine protocol for acute acetaminophen intoxication. *Clin Ther.* 2005 Mar;27(3):336–41.

13. Lauterburg BH, Corcoran GB, Mitchell JR. Mechanism of action of N-acetylcysteine in the protection against the hepatotoxicity of acetaminophen in rats in vivo. *J Clin Invest.* 1983 Apr;71(4):980–91.

14. Prescott LF, Park J, Ballantyne A, Adriaenssens P, Proudfoot AT. Treatment of paracetamol (acetaminophen) poisoning with N-acetylcysteine. *Lancet.* 1977 Aug 27;2(8035):432–4.

15. Ghirlanda G, Oradei A, Manto A, et al. Evidence of plasma CoQ10-lowering effect by HMG-CoA reductase inhibitors: a double-blind, placebo-controlled study. *J Clin Pharmacol.* 1993 Mar;33(3):226–9.

16. Moling O, Cairon E, Rimenti G, Rizza F, Pristerá R, Mian P. Severe hepatotoxicity after therapeutic doses of acetaminophen. *Clin Ther.* 2006 May;28(5):755–60.

17. Bolesta S, Haber SL. Hepatotoxicity associated with chronic acetaminophen administration in patients without risk factors. *Ann Pharmacother.* 2002 Feb;36(2):331–3.

18. Chun LJ, Tong MJ, Busuttil RW, Hiatt JR. Acetaminophen hepatotoxicity and acute liver failure. *J Clin Gastroenterol.* 2009 Apr;43(4):342–9.

19. Lee WM. Acetaminophen and the US Acute liver failure study group: lowering the risks of hepatic failure. *Hepatology.* 2004 Jul;40(1):6–9.

20. Watkins PB, Kaplowitz N, Slattery JT, et al. Aminotransferase elevations in healthy adults receiving 4 grams of acetaminophen daily: a randomized controlled trial. *JAMA.* 2006 Jul 5;296(1):87–93.

21. Bonkovsky HL, Kane RE, Jones DP, Galinsky RE, Banner B. Acute hepatic and renal toxicity from low doses of acetaminophen in the absence of alcohol abuse or malnutrition: evidence for increased susceptibility to drug toxicity due to cardiopulmonary and renal insufficiency. *Hepatology.* 1994 May;19(5):1141–8.

22. Blakely P, McDonald BR. Acute renal failure due to acetaminophen ingestion: a case report and review of the literature. *J Am Soc Nephrol.* 1995 Jul;6(1):48–53.

23. Zaffanello M, Brugnara M, Angeli S, Cuzzolin L. Acute non-oliguric kidney failure and cholestatic hepatitis induced by ibuprofen and acetaminophen: a case report. *Acta Paediatr.* 2009 May;98(5):903–5.

24. Björck S, Svalander CT, Aurell M. Acute renal failure after analgesic drugs including paracetamol (acetaminophen). *Nephron.* 1988; 49(1):45–53.

25. Gago-Dominguez M, Yuan JM, Castelao JE, Ross RK, Yu MC. Regular use of analgesics is a risk factor for renal cell carcinoma. *Br J Cancer.* 1999 Oct;81(3):542–8.

26. McLaughlin JK, Blot WJ, Mehl ES, Fraumeni JF Jr. Relation of analgesic use to renal cancer: population-based findings. *Natl Cancer Inst Monogr.* 1985 Dec;69:217–22.

27. Derby LE, Jick H. Acetaminophen and renal and bladder cancer. *Epidemiology.* 1996 Jul;7(4):358–62.

28. Kaye JA, Myers MW, Jick H. Acetaminophen and the risk of renal and bladder cancer in the general practice research database. *Epidemiology.* 2001 Nov;12(6):690–4.

29. Price LM, Poklis A, Johnson DE. Fatal acetaminophen poisoning with evidence of subendocardial necrosis of the heart. *J Forensic Sci.* 1991 May;36(3):930–5.

30. Nourjah P, Ahmad SR, Karwoski C, Willy M. Estimates of acetaminophen (Paracetamol)-associated overdoses in the United States. *Pharmacoepidemiol Drug Saf.* 2006 Jun;15(6):398–405.

31. Available at: http://www.kidney-cancer- symptoms.com. Accessed April 14, 2010.

32. Derby LE, Jick H. Acetaminophen and renal and bladder cancer. *Epidemiology.* 1996 Jul;7(4):358–62.

33. Kaye JA, Myers MW, Jick H. Acetaminophen and the risk of renal and bladder cancer in the general practice research database. *Epidemiology.* 2001 Nov;12(6):690–4.

34. Pantuck AJ, Zisman A, Belldegrun AS. The changing natural history of renal cell carcinoma. *J Urol.* 2001 Nov;166(5):1611–23.

35. Qian W, Shichi H. Acetaminophen produces cataract in DBA2 mice by Ah receptor-independent induction of CYP1A2. *J Ocul Pharmacol Ther*. 2000 Aug;16(4):337–44.

36. Available at: http://www.nlm.nih.gov/medlineplus/ency/article/002598.htm. Accessed July 30, 2009.

37. Garcia Rodríguez LA, Hernández-Díaz S. The risk of upper gastrointestinal complications associated with nonsteroidal anti-inflammatory drugs, glucocorticoids, acetaminophen, and combinations of these agents. *Arthritis Res*. 2001; 3(2):98–101.

38. Beasley R, Clayton T, Crane J, et al. Association between paracetamol use in infancy and childhood, and risk of asthma, rhinoconjunctivitis, and eczema in children aged 6–7 years: analysis from Phase Three of the ISAAC programme. *Lancet*. 2008 Sep 20;372(9643):1039–48.

39. Lawyer AB. Paracetamol as a risk factor for allergic disorders. *Lancet*. 2009 Jan 10;373(9658):121.

40. Forman JP, Stampfer MJ, Curhan GC. Non-narcotic analgesic dose and risk of incident hypertension in US women. *Hypertension*. 2005 Sep;46(3):500–7.

41. Rathbun WB, Killen CE, Holleschau AM, Nagasawa HT. Maintenance of hepatic glutathione homeostasis and prevention of acetaminophen-induced cataract in mice by L-cysteine prodrugs. *Biochem Pharmacol*. 1996 May 3;51(9):1111–6.

42. Zhao C, Shichi H. Prevention of acetaminophen-induced cataract by a combination of diallyl disulfide and N-acetylcysteine. J Ocul *Pharmacol Ther*. 1998 Aug;14(4):345–55.

43. Available at: http://www.cnn.com/2009/HEALTH/06/30/acetaminophen.fda.hearing/. Accessed July 20, 2009.

44. Available at: http://www.fda.gov/NewsEvents/Newsroom/PressAnnouncements/ucm149573.htm. Accessed July 20, 2009.

45. Available at: http://abcnews.go.com/Health/PainManagement/Story?id=7965902&page=1. Accessed July 20, 2009.

46. Available at: http://www.drugs.com/news/acetaminophen-hazardous-hepatitis-1807.html. Accessed July 20, 2009.

47. Available at: http://www.fda.gov/ohrms/dockets/ac/02/ transcripts/3882T1.htm. Accessed July 20, 2009.

48. Available at: http://www.msnbc.msn.com/id/4031091. Accessed July 27, 2009.

49. Available at: http://www.fda.gov/downloads/Drugs/Drug-Safety/InformationbyDrugClass/UCM171901.pd. Accessed July 27, 2009.

50. Piper JM, Tonascia J, Matanoski GM. Heavy phenacetin use and bladder cancer in women aged 20 to 49 years. N Engl J Med. 1985 Aug;313(5):292-5.

51. Unet MS, ChowWH, McLaughiin K, et al. Analgesics and cancers of the renal pelvis and ureter. Int J Cancer. 1995 Jul 4;62(11):15-8.

52. McCredie M, Stewart H, Day NE. Different roles for phenacetin and paracetamol in cancer of the kidney and renal pelvis. Int J Cancer. 1993 Jan 21;(5312):245-9.

53. Brunner FR, Selwood NH. End-stage renal failure due to analgesic nephropathy. Its changing pattern and cardiovascular mortality. Nephrol Dial Transplant. 1994; 9(10):1371-6.

54. Stewart JH, Hobbs JB, McCredie MB. Morphologic evidence that analgesic-induced kidney pathology contributes to the progression of tumors of the renal pelvis. Cancer. 1999 Oct 15;86(8):1576-82.

55. Leventhal LJ, Boyce EG, Zurier RB. Treatment of rheumatoid arthritis with gammalinolenic acid. Ann Intern Med. 1993 Nov 1;119(9):867-73.

56. Fortin PR, Lew RA, Liang MH, et al. Validation of a meta-analysis: the effects of fish oil in rheumatoid arthritis. J Clin Epidemiol. 1995 Nov;48(11):1379-90.

57. Kremer JM, Lawrence DA, Petrillo GF, et al. Effects of high-dose fish oil on rheumatoid arthritis after stopping nonsteroidal antiinflammatory drugs. Clinical and immune correlates. Arthritis Rheum. 1995 Aug;38(8):1107-14.

58. Kim LS, Axelrod LJ, Howard P, Buratovich N, Waters RF. Efficacy of methylsulfonylmethane (MSM) in osteoarthritis pain of the knee: a pilot clinical trial. Osteoarthritis Cartilage. 2006 Mar;14(3):286-94.

59. Usha PR, Naidu MU. Randomised, double-blind, parallel, placebo-controlled study of oral glucosamine, methylsulfonylmethane and their combination in osteoarthritis. *Clin Drug Investig.* 2004; 24(6):353–63.

60. Choi SS, Han KJ, Lee JK, et al. Antinociceptive mechanisms of orally administered decursinol in the mouse. *Life Sci.* 2003 Jun 13;73(4):471–85.

61. Choi SS, Han KJ, Lee HK, Han EJ, Suh HW. Antinociceptive profiles of crude extract from roots of Angelica gigas NAKAI in various pain models. *Biol Pharm Bull.* 2003 Sep;26(9):1283–8.

How Much More FDA *Abuse* Can Americans Tolerate?

I HAVE EXPOSED SO MANY HORRIFIC SCANDALS within the FDA that even I thought the agency couldn't get any worse. I thought wrong!

At the heart of the FDA's rationale for existence is its supposed ability to evaluate findings from human clinical drug trials. The FDA's ultimate decision to approve or reject a new drug is based on how the drug performs in human trials.

If you ever wonder why a drug works so well in clinical trials, but then inflicts lethal side effects (and only mediocre efficacy) after FDA approval, one part of the answer is that the clinical trials themselves are often fraudulent.[1–9]

In a revelation widely reported by the news media, a crooked clinic helped conduct 170 drug studies for nearly every major pharmaceutical company and routinely falsified data and patient records. The clinic's criminal conduct rendered the findings from the human trials they conducted meaningless. The FDA relied on these fraudulent findings, however, to approve drugs used by tens of millions of Americans.[10]

FDA LETS CRIMINALS OVERSEE CLINICAL TRIALS

The shocker is that after federal agents raided this clinic and those who perpetrated these illegal acts pleaded guilty to fraud, the FDA did not ban them from participating in additional human clinical drug trials![11]

According to federal law, the FDA had five years from the criminal conviction to ban the perpetrators from conducting further drug research. In this case, the FDA did nothing for over four years, and then sent the revocation notice to the wrong address. The result is that those involved in these criminal acts are free to continue conducting human clinical trials.[12]

When Congress learned of the FDA's gross incompetence, they conducted their usual hearings in which FDA officials are subpoenaed to appear before a Congressional oversight committee to explain how such a blatant error could occur.

Congressional investigators found the FDA pays little attention to its responsibilities to ban researchers convicted of fraud and is totally disorganized about carrying out revocation procedures.[13]

The General Accounting Office reviewed 18 instances of research fraud and found the FDA took between one and 11 years to ban these criminals. FDA negligence enabled those convicted of fraud to conduct human experimentation for years.[12,14] Is it any wonder why so many FDA-approved drugs kill their users either from side effects or lack of efficacy?

THE URGENT NEED FOR RADICAL FDA REFORM

If radical FDA reform is not enacted, most people reading this article will suffer premature aging and death.

This book *Pharmocracy* provides a plethora of irrefutable facts that provide Congress with a basis to radically reform the FDA so as to remove its compulsory and incompetent dictatorial power to prevent Americans from accessing safe medications.

References

1. Available at: http://firstclinical.com/journal/2007/0701_Fraud.pdf. Accessed April 8, 2011.

2. Available at: http://www.naturalnews.com/001298.html. Accessed April 8, 2011.

3. Available at: http://www.drugsettlement.com/articles/ketek-linked-liver-failure-drug-company-doctor-convicted-fraud. Accessed April 8, 2011.

4. Available at: http://oig.hhs.gov/publications/docs/press/2007/FDAClinicalTrials3.pdf. Accessed April 8, 2011.

5. Available at: http://pn.psychiatryonline.org/content/39/13/1.1.full. Accessed April 8, 2011.

6. Available at: http://www.biospace.com/news_story.aspx?NewsEntityId=130116. Accessed April 8, 2011.

7. Available at: http://blogs.wsj.com/health/2010/01/15/feds-accuse-doc-of-faking-research-on-pfizer-merck-drugs/. Accessed April 8, 2011.

8. Available at: http://www.guardian.co.uk/business/2004/jun/03/mentalhealth.medicineandhealth. Accessed April 8, 2011.

9. Available at: http://online.wsj.com/article/SB123672510903888207.html?mod=googlenews_wsj. Accessed April 8, 2011.

10. Available at: http://www.nytimes.com/1999/05/17/business/a-doctor-s-drug-trials-turn-into-fraud.html. Accessed April 8, 2011.

11. Available at: http://www.nytimes.com/2009/10/22/health/
    policy/22fda.html?_r=1. Accessed April 8, 2011.

12. Available at: http://www.naturalnews.com/027536_criminals_
    doctors.html. Accessed April 8, 2011.

13. Available at: http://www.nytimes.com/2006/04/24/
    washington/24fda.html?fta=y. Accessed April 8, 2011.

14. Available at: http://online.wsj.com/article/SB125622345164801405.
    html. Accessed April 8, 2011.

Drug Company Pleads Guilty to Health Fraud

L IFE EXTENSION® HAS SPENT the last three decades exposing horrific financial and scientific fraud perpetrated by the pharmaceutical industry and the FDA.

We have revealed how pervasive pharmaceutical deceit infiltrates government, academia, and the media, causing consumers to pay outrageous prices for dangerous drugs that provide little or no benefit.

In an unprecedented development, a pharmaceutical giant has pled guilty to a felony with the intent to defraud, and its parent has agreed to pay a record $2.3 billion to reimburse Medicare, Medicaid, and other agencies for drugs that were marketed in violation of various federal laws.[1]

For those who labor under the misconception that pharmaceutical companies serve benevolent purposes, the multiple criminal counts you are about to read will eradicate this fallacy.

LETHAL DRUG ILLEGALLY PROMOTED AT HIGHER THAN ALLOWED DOSES

Most of you are familiar with the Vioxx® scandal, in which pharmaceutical giant Merck has spent billions of dollars defending and settling lawsuits showing that the deadly dangers of this drug were known long *before* it was withdrawn.

A lesser-known arthritis drug in this category called Bextra® was also withdrawn because of increased risks of heart attacks and strokes, as well as deaths, in patients for whom it was prescribed it.[2–4]

In a startling admission, a subsidiary of pharmaceutical behemoth Pfizer has pled guilty to a criminal charge that it fraudulently sold Bextra® not to treat arthritis, but to be used in higher doses to relieve acute surgical pain.[5]

Even at the usual dose, Bextra® inflicted fatal side effects. In a 2004 analysis presented at the American Heart Association, Bextra® was shown to more than double the risk of heart attack or stroke. The lead author of this study commented, that "This is a time bomb waiting to go off."[6]

The record financial payout by Pfizer is not the result of the fact that Bextra® injured or killed arthritis patients. It is, rather, to settle government claims that Pfizer illegally promoted the sale of Bextra® for uses and dosages that the FDA specifically declined to approve due to safety concerns. Of the total settlement, $1.195 billion represents a fine for the fraudulent marketing of Bextra®—the largest criminal fine ever imposed in the United States for any matter.

LIFE EXTENSION® MEMBERS LEARNED OF THESE DANGERS YEARS EARLIER

Years before the public learned about the dangers of Vioxx® and Bextra®, the Life Extension Foundation® warned its members that these drugs would create lethal havoc in the body.

The reason is that by selectively blocking the cyclooxygenase-2 (COX-2) enzyme, an imbalance is created that results in increased amounts of thromboxane A2 and leukotriene B4 being produced.[7-9]

Thromboxane A2 promotes abnormal arterial blood clots, the leading cause of acute heart attack and stroke.[10] Leukotriene B4 inflicts massive inflammatory damage to the arterial wall and other tissues of the body.[11]

COX-2 inhibiting drugs like Vioxx® and Bextra® can increase thromboxane A2 and leukotriene B4, unless healthy dietary changes are instituted. This means reducing or eliminating from one's diet arachidonic acid-rich foods (egg yolk, red meat, poultry, and dairy), high-glycemic index carbohydrates, and omega-6 fats. The adverse effects of COX-2 inhibiting drugs may also be mitigated by taking a low-dose aspirin tablet each day, along with fish oil and curcumin.[12-14]

Based on these deadly underlying mechanisms, Life Extension® knew that Vioxx®, Bextra®, and other drugs in this category would kill thousands of unsuspecting patients. Arrayed against us were pharmaceutical companies that spent billions of dollars misleading consumers and doctors into believing these drugs were "safer" than aspirin.

We don't believe the government even realizes how many needless deaths may have occurred as a result of the unauthorized and illegal promotion of Bextra®. The government focused its criminal charges instead on paperwork violations and financial losses to Medicare and Medicaid, not the patients injured by the illegal sale of this lethal drug.

CASH KICKBACKS PAID TO DOCTORS
TO PRESCRIBE DRUGS

Part of the $2.3 billion settlement involves allegations that Pfizer paid doctors kickbacks to induce them to prescribe the following drugs:

Drug	Indication
Aricept®	Alzheimer's
Celebrex®	Arthritis
Lipitor®	High Cholesterol and LDL
Norvasc®	Hypertension
Relpax®	Migraine
Viagra®	Impotence
Zithromax®	Antibiotic
Zoloft®	Depression
Zyrtec®	Allergy

The government's complaint describes how Pfizer compensated doctors to prescribe these drugs in some instances by providing cash payments, or so-called "gifts," such as travel, entertainment, and meals. Illegal remuneration was also allegedly paid to doctors in the form of speaker fees, mentorships, preceptorships, and journal clubs.

When one reviews the diverse list of drugs that Pfizer is claimed to have paid doctors to prescribe, it is no wonder they grew to become the largest pharmaceutical company in the world.

PHYSICIANS PAID TO ILLEGALLY PRESCRIBE DRUGS

It's one thing to break the law by paying doctors to prescribe drugs that at least have some degree of documented efficacy, but Pfizer went further than this.

The government's complaint describes how Pfizer created new uses for its patented drugs and then engaged in all kinds of devious schemes to illegally promote these "new uses" to physicians. For instance, Pfizer claimed its drug Lyrica® was superior to lower-cost generic medications that treat neuropathic and surgical pain, and then illegally compensated doctors to prescribe Lyrica® for these indications.[15]

Geodon® is a drug approved to treat schizophrenia or acute bipolar mania, but the government outlined in its complaint that Pfizer was inappropriately and illegally promoting it for use in children and adults to treat autism, attention deficit hyperactivity disorder, mood disorders, and depression. The government contended that Pfizer illegally promoted Geodon® at dosages that were off-label and "offered and paid illegal remuneration to healthcare professionals to induce them to promote and prescribe Geodon® in violation of the Federal Anti-Kickback Statute."[16]

Zyvox® is an antibiotic Pfizer makes to treat deadly antibiotic-resistant MRSA staph infections. The settlement agreement outlined various alleged misconduct relating to the illegal marketing of this drug, including how Pfizer falsely advertised that Zyvox® was superior to generic vancomycin and then illegally paid doctors to prescribe it.[17]

PFIZER GETS BY WITH A SLAP ON THE WRIST

In the settlement agreement, Pfizer only has to agree to admit to the Bextra® criminal charge. In exchange for paying a total of $2.3 billion, Pfizer is allowed to claim a denial of the government's other allegations.

To give you an idea what a drop in the bucket this payout is to Pfizer, when a one-time tax break was given to corporations that repatriated offshore profits, Pfizer brought back $37 billion of cash stashed away from its foreign operations.[18] Pfizer did this because the tax rate was only 5.25% that year. Considering how much more they made in their largest market (the United States), writing a $2.3 billion check to settle these massive fraud claims is pocket change to a company the size of Pfizer.

This is not the first time Pfizer was caught committing these illegal acts. Prosecutors noted that this was Pfizer's fourth such settlement since 2002.[1] In fact, according to the US Attorney, while Pfizer was negotiating deals over past misconduct, they were continuing to violate the same laws with other drugs.[19]

Contrast Pfizer's "slap-on-the-wrist" fine to what the FDA does to those who practice alternative medicine. Under far less egregious circumstances, the government seizes everything owned by alternative practitioners and often threatens harsh jail sentences.

DRUG COMPANIES PAY GHOSTWRITERS

According to a study released by editors of the *Journal of the American Medical Association*, drug companies pay doctors with prestigious university affiliations to put their name on so-called "scientific papers" that are written by ghostwriters.[20]

These pharmaceutical company-financed articles, carefully calibrated to sell expensive prescription drugs, slip by the peer-review process and make it into the top medical journals. Not only do these articles influence physicians' prescribing practices, but they are often picked up by the media, which then runs favorable news articles about these deceptively promoted drugs.

As Life Extension® reported last year, the drug company Wyeth faces 8,400 lawsuits from women who claim Premarin® or PremPro® caused them to become ill. Court documents from these cases reveal that Wyeth paid ghost-writers to produce 26 "scientific" papers supporting the use of their dangerous female hormone drugs.[21]

The Wyeth-funded articles extolled purported benefits of these unnatural hormone drugs while downplaying their lethal risks. Nowhere in these articles was Wyeth's role in initiating and paying for them disclosed.

Court documents show how Wyeth contracted with private companies to outline articles, draft them, and then solicit top physicians to sign their names, even though many of the doctors contributed little or no writing to them. These tainted articles were published in medical journals between 1998 and 2005, and helped generate billions of dollars of sales for Wyeth.[21]

The latest corroboration of large-scale drug company-induced ghostwriting substantiates what Life Extension® uncovered decades ago: drug companies manipulate scientific data to deceive doctors into prescribing dangerous drugs.

If you wonder how pharmaceutical companies have been able to defraud the American public for so many decades, look no further than the incestuous relationship they maintain with the FDA. By providing the pharmaceutical industry a virtual monopoly over drug sales in the United States, as the FDA does, consumers have only limited options when they contract a serious illness.

Those who offer alternatives to FDA-approved drugs often find themselves under criminal or civil investigation by any number of federal agencies, thus impeding or outright blocking their ability to compete against pharmaceutical behemoths.

References

1. Available at: http://www.miamiherald.com/101/story/1216716. html. Accessed October 21, 2009.

2. Available at: http://www.medicinenet.com/script/main/art. asp?articlekey=46601. Accessed October 21, 2009.

3. Roumie CL, Mitchel EF Jr, Kaltenbach L, Arbogast PG, Gideon P, Griffin MR. Nonaspirin NSAIDs, cyclooxygenase 2 inhibitors, and the risk for stroke. *Stroke.* 2008 Jul;39(7):2037–45.

4. Roumie CL, Choma NN, Kaltenbach L, Mitchel EF Jr, Arbogast PG, Griffin MR. Non-aspirin NSAIDs, cyclooxygenase-2 inhibitors and risk for cardiovascular events-stroke, acute myocardial infarction, and death from coronary heart disease. *Pharmacoepidemiol Drug Saf.* 2009 Nov;18(11):1053–63.

5. Available at: http://online.wsj.com/article/ SB125190160702979723.html. Accessed October 21, 2009.

6. Available at: http://www.medscape.com/viewarticle/538008. Accessed October 21, 2009.

7. Khanapure SP, Garvey DS, Janero DR, Letts LG. Eicosanoids in inflammation: biosynthesis, pharmacology, and therapeutic frontiers. *Curr Top Med Chem.* 2007;7(3):311–40.

8. Mao JT, Tsu IH, Dubinett SM, et al. Modulation of pulmonary leukotriene B4 production by cyclooxygenase-2 inhibitors and lipopolysaccharide. *Clin Cancer Res.* 2004 Oct 15;10(20):6872–8.

9. Snyderman CH, Abbas MM, Wagner R, D'Amico F. Inhibition of growth of a murine squamous cell carcinoma by a cyclooxygenase inhibitor increases leukotriene B4 production. *Arch Otolaryngol Head Neck Surg.* 1995 Sep;121(9):1017–20.

10. Cheng Y, Austin SC, Rocca B, et al. Role of prostacyclin in the cardiovascular response to thromboxane A2. *Science.* 2002 Apr 19;296(5567):539–41.

11. Subbarao K, Jala VR, Mathis S, et al. Role of leukotriene B4 receptors in the development of atherosclerosis: potential mechanisms. *Arterioscler Thromb Vasc Biol.* 2004 Feb;24(2):369–75.

12. Leaberry BA. Aspirin for the prevention of cardiovascular disease: systematic review. *J Nurs Care Qual.* 2010 Jan-Mar;25(1):17–21.

13. Lavie CJ, Milani RV, Mehra MR, Ventura HO. Omega-3 poly-unsaturated fatty acids and cardiovascular diseases. *J Am Coll Cardiol.* 2009 Aug 11;54(7):585–94.

14. Srivastava G, Mehta JL. Currying the heart: curcumin and cardioprotection. J Cardiovasc *Pharmacol Ther.* 2009 Mar;14(1):22–7.

15. Available at: http://www.ahrp.org/cms/content/view/633/9/. Accessed October 28, 2009.

16. Available at: http://www.justice.gov/usao/pae/News/Pr/2009/sep/pfizerrelease.pdf Accessed October 28, 2009.

17. Available at: http://www.reuters.com/article/pressRelease/idUS160827+02-Sep-2009+PRN20090902. Accessed October 28, 2009.

18. Available at: http://www.nytimes.com/2008/06/24/business/24tax.html. Accessed October 28, 2009.

19. Available at: http://www.msnbc.msn.com/id/32657347/ns/business-us_business/. Accessed October 28, 2009.

20. Ross JS, Hill KP, Egilman DS, Krumholz HM. Guest author-ship and ghostwriting in publications related to rofecoxib: a case study of industry documents from rofecoxib litigation. *JAMA.* 2008 Apr 16;299(15):1800–12.

21. Available at: http://www.nytimes.com/2009/08/05/health/research/05ghost.html. Accessed October 29, 2009.

2009

Why American Healthcare is Headed for Collapse

W HILE POLITICIANS DEBATE a wide range of financial issues, the most dangerous threat to the United States economy is ignored as if it did not exist. The reason you don't hear about this problem is that no one seems to know how to solve it.

I will briefly review this impending disaster and then provide some real world solutions. For the benefit of new members, the Life Extension Foundation® predicted today's healthcare cost crisis back in the early 1980s. Our prophetic warnings were ridiculed at the time, but events over the past decade document the financial train wreck we fought so hard to prevent.

Discussions rage today about how to provide universal healthcare. Overlooked is the fact that the government will soon be unable to pay the medical costs it is already on the hook for. Not only do 40 million Americans depend

on these government-funded programs, but these individuals have already paid for them with their Medicare
tax dollars.

THE MAGNITUDE OF THIS ISSUE

Very soon, Medicare will start paying out more in hospital bills than the premiums (taxes) it will collect. When
that time arrives, the federal government will have to tap
some other source to cover this gargantuan unfunded liability. One obstacle is that the federal government is over
$11 trillion in debt and is projected to run trillion dollar
deficits for the next several years. If these numbers sound
high, they pale in comparison to Medicare's unfunded liability of $34 trillion.

To put this in perspective, the government collects only
about $2 trillion each year in total tax revenue (including
Medicare premium taxes).[1] There are virtually no reserve
funds left to pay promised Medicare (and Medicaid) benefits. The government is relying on the money it takes in
each day to cover its enormous Medicare cost burden.

As the country ages, Medicare will devour huge chunks
of US economic output and eventually overwhelm every
other item on the federal budget. While politicians stick
their heads in the sand and disregard this issue, no one
can argue against the math showing a financial disaster of
unprecedented magnitude.

MEDICARE SCAMS

The government points to rampant fraud as one reason
behind Medicare problems. It is estimated that 20% of
every dollar Medicare pays out goes to criminals who submit claims for nonexistent or bogus services. For example,
it was recently discovered that Medicare paid out $100

million for wheelchairs, canes, prescription drugs, and other items prescribed by dead doctors.[2] In other words, people working at doctor's offices pretended their doctors never died and falsely billed Medicare for medical treatments that were never rendered.

The government brags when it cracks down on Medicare fraud, but they only catch a fraction of the crimes perpetrated. The reality is that the living con artists defraud Medicare out of far more than dead doctors do.

What the government does not like to admit is that another 20% of Medicare dollars are paid out in the form of overpayments to those with political connections. What companies do is lobby Congress to enact legislation mandating that Medicare pay inflated prices for certain products and services that can be obtained for a fraction of the price on the free market. This enables those who are politically connected to grossly overcharge Medicare because Congress mandates the inflated expenditures.

How inflated are the monies Medicare pays out? Take for example, an oxygen concentrator, a device that delivers oxygen through a tube to patients with respiratory illness. You can buy one new on the open market for $600. By law, Medicare is only allowed to rent these devices at a price that winds up costing $7,142 over a 36-month period. Medicare covers 80%, so it spends $5,714, while the patient has to pay the other 20%, or $1,428.[3] Under this absurd system, Medicare and patients can pay ten times the free market price it would cost to buy the device new! (Think how much money would be saved if the devices were bought used?)

Perhaps the most expensive politically-induced overcharge is for prescription drugs. Under the Medicare Prescription Drug Act that Life Extension® vehemently battled against, Medicare is required by law to pay full retail drug prices.[4]

The Medicare Prescription Drug Act was largely written by pharmaceutical companies and passed under intense pressure by pharmaceutical lobbyists (refer to the August 2007 issue of *Life Extension Magazine®* for the sordid details).[5] Medicare will pay out hundreds of billions of dollars for drugs that could be obtained for far less in a competitive-bidding system, something that the Medicare Prescription Drug Act prohibits.

THE GENERIC DRUG RIP OFF

Once a brand drug comes off patent, generic equivalents emerge, but they cost far more than they need to because of FDA overregulation.

Take the drug finasteride (Proscar®), for example. It came off patent in the year 2006, but at the end of 2008 chain pharmacies were charging about $90 for 30 tablets (a one-month supply). All it takes to make this drug is to put 5 mg of finasteride into a tablet that dissolves in the stomach. Vitamin companies do this every day with nutrients, but the FDA does not allow them to freely do the same thing with drugs.

We checked on the cost of buying finasteride and making it into tablets. The free market price for 30 tablets is only $10.25, which includes independent assay of the ingredient quality, potency and tablet dissolution—and a reasonable profit margin. It is against the law, however, for GMP-certified (Good Manufacturing Practices) vitamin manufacturers to be able to offer low-cost generic drugs. This prohibition must be lifted as America can no longer afford to subsidize those who are politically connected while the country is driven into insolvency.

Finasteride is a drug that not only helps relieve benign prostate enlargement, but that may also reduce the risk prostate cancer.[7-9] Widespread use could save Medicare lots of money in expensive prostate treatments. Those who follow *Life Extension*'s other recommendations would be expected to reduce prostate cancer risk even more.

As evidence mounts about the prostate cancer risk reduction associated with drugs like finasteride, more companies are competing to make it, but its average price at chain pharmacies is around $86 a month—a staggering eight times higher than what its free market price would be!

Please note that generic prices tend to wildly fluctuate. In this case, as more competitors entered the market, chain pharmacies did not substantially lower the price of finasteride. In some cases, the opposite occurred, and by the time you read this, the price could be different.

MEDICARE PAYS FOR HIV TREATMENTS NEVER DELIVERED

It is remarkable how creative people get when a bloated government bureaucracy such as Medicare/Medicaid pays out almost $500 billion each year with few questions asked.

According to the federal government, hundreds of Medicare-licensed clinics in South Florida defraud Medicare with fake HIV-drug claims. The scam is not hard to pull off. Clinics find indigent HIV-infected drug users who agree to "sell" their cards to the clinics and pretend they are receiving outrageously expensive HIV infusion treatments. These kinds of therapies were long ago abandoned in favor of more effective antiviral drugs, but Medicare pays for them anyway.

To give you an idea of the magnitude of the problem, just one drug addict enabled one clinic to file more than $1.1

million in false Medicare claims for these fabricated anti-HIV infusions.[6]

Even if these treatments were medically necessary, they would only be needed once or twice a month. In one instance, scammers billed Medicare three times a day for each patient—and Medicare paid these bills! According to the federal officials, Medicare continued to pay these clinics for multiple HIV infusion treatments (costing $1,500 to $3,000 per therapy) because Medicare allows them.

THE REAL PROBLEM

Despite inappropriate disbursements that Medicare makes based on private sector fraud and political corruption, the main culprit behind Medicare's eminent collapse is the demographics.

Like Social Security (which is nowhere near as broke as Medicare), the federal government forced workers to pay premiums (taxes) for their Medicare "insurance." Private insurance companies are required by law to maintain reserves in order to pay out future claims. The federal government, on the other hand, has been running a Ponzi scheme and has exhausted virtually every penny. The government is now on the hook for $34 trillion of liabilities. No one knows where the money will come from for these future Medicare/Medicaid disbursements.

A VERY RADICAL APPROACH

I am as libertarian in my thinking as anyone I know, but there are radical approaches that could not only spare Medicare, but protect future generations as well.

Cigarettes officially kill 440,000 people in the US each year, but the real number is higher. When tabulating cigarette smoking-induced deaths, many cancers related to cigarette smoking (such as pancreatic and esophageal cancers) are not always counted.[23]

The fact that 18-year-olds are allowed to buy something as addictive as cigarettes is obscene. What is worse is that even if a person stops smoking in their 20s, the DNA gene damage inflicted in their early years predisposes them to lifelong increased cancer risks.

I am personally livid over the amount of secondhand smoke I was forced to inhale throughout my early life. It could very well be the cause of my death.

While outright prohibition would not work in the long term, the federal government could impose a three-month moratorium on all tobacco sales. This would enable a huge number of smokers to quit. Financial penalties for anyone caught selling cigarettes during this proposed three-month ban could be so large that it might conceivably work.

If just 30% of all smokers stopped as a result of this three-month moratorium, that alone might save Medicare. Just debating it in Congress may remind smokers of what they are doing to their bodies and motivate them to break their addiction.

I realize this proposal is draconian and would be still another government intrusion on individual liberty. The facts, however, are that smoking-related illnesses are responsible for a huge portion of Medicare/Medicaid outlays—and this country can no longer afford it.

PARTIAL SOLUTIONS

If you are curious as to why Congress has failed so miserably in overseeing Medicare, look no further than the political contributions and lobbying efforts made by those who benefit by scamming the Medicare system. Partial reform will happen when free market forces are allowed to compete for

Medicare dollars, as opposed to the bureaucratic albatross that now exists.

One problem is that Medicare will only pay for FDA-approved medical devices and drugs. As we know, this means that Medicare recipients are forced into overpriced therapies that are laden with side effects. Treating drug-induced side effects results in the expenditure of even more healthcare dollars. To make matters worse, the efficacy of certain FDA-approved drugs is so mediocre that patients sometimes live only a few months longer by taking them. The cost to Medicare for these drugs can easily exceed $50,000 per patient. Complementary physicians who prescribe unapproved cancer therapies that cost a fraction of FDA-approved drugs are subject to criminal prosecution.

So we have a system in place today in which progressive doctors are persecuted, while those who sell dangerous and often ineffective therapies receive protection and payment from the federal government. People without the financial wherewithal have no choice, since Medicare will only pay for what the FDA claims is safe and effective. Conventional medicine's goldmine will end when Medicare exhausts its ability to pay.

A group of FDA scientists recently revolted against their superiors and went directly to Congress.[10] The reason was that they were told by their superiors to certify new medical devices as safe and effective, when the clinical testing data showed the opposite. This is just one example of how the FDA contributes to today's healthcare cost crisis by allowing dangerous products on to the market that Medicare then pays for.

ONE WAY TO SLASH MEDICARE OUTLAYS

Low blood levels of vitamin D are associated with increased incidences of virtually every human disease.[11–14]

In 2007, I petitioned the federal government to mandate vitamin D supplementation in Medicare-eligible individuals in order for them to be eligible to receive benefits.[15] I proposed that the government require that people must have a minimum blood level of 32 ng/mL of vitamin D or they would be denied coverage. This would force aging people to take this ultra-low-cost supplement, which in turn would drastically slash the incidences of the most common aging-related disorders.

Optimal vitamin D blood levels are over 50 ng/mL, yet most Americans' levels test far below 30.[16–19] By mandating basic vitamin D supplementation, Medicare might regain some of its solvency, as it would be paying out far fewer medical expenses.

A study published in the *New England Journal of Medicine* evaluated blood levels for vitamin D in intensive care unit (ICU) patients.[20] The average serum vitamin D level was only 16 ng/mL. All patients with undetectable levels of vitamin D died.

Patients with the lowest vitamin D blood levels had the most severe organ dysfunction and the most adverse outcomes. The predicted mortality (death) rate was:

Vitamin D Status	Mortality Percentage
ICU patients with sufficient vitamin D	16%
ICU patients with insufficient vitamin D	35%
ICU patients with deficient vitamin D	45%

It costs Medicare about $2,674 a day to care for ICU patients, and some of them linger for weeks or months in

this expensive hospital setting.[21] Mandating optimal vitamin D levels could slash the number of Medicare patients
requiring ICU care.

HARSH REALITIES

While common sense solutions exist, the aging population
will challenge the solvency of Medicare unless something
radical is done to keep humans healthy.

Mainstream medicine bases its financial projections on
lots of aging people contracting cancer, vascular disease,
and dementia. Today's medicinal "industry" does not want
any interference with their income stream and have no
incentive to institute preventive programs.

The public is more health conscious today than ever. The
problem is that too many people continue to abuse their
bodies with excess intake of dangerous calories, cigarette
smoking, and physical inactivity. Add to this the insufficient intake of nutrients such as magnesium, vitamin D,
omega-3s, and it is no wonder that healthcare expenditures are bankrupting this country.[22]

GOVERNMENT HAS TO FESS UP TO THE PROBLEM

To shock the public into a pro-active state, the federal government has to admit that they are not able to pay future
Medicare claims unless aggressive steps are taken to prevent age-related disease. The public needs to know that if
they don't take personal responsibility for their healthcare, there may be no Medicare dollars available to cover
their sick care.

The government needs to initiate mandatory warnings
(that I would be happy to write) on the labels of all dangerous foods. People would be less likely to buy toxic foods if
they were reminded about the risks associated with eating

them. The government should encourage food companies to state truthful claims about healthy foods such as "eating broccoli reduces cancer risk."

The main reason Medicare is facing insolvency is that too many aging people are getting sick. These diseases of aging are preventable via a wide variety of lifestyle alterations. It will require a sustained governmental public relations campaign to hammer in the need for Americans to follow healthier lifestyles.

Alternatively, lifting the ban currently in place that precludes the dissemination of truthful health information about a wide variety of foods, hormones, nutrients, and even certain drugs would make a significant positive impact on the aging population, which in turn would help resolve the catastrophic Medicare cost crisis we now face.

IMPORTANT UPDATE

In the January 2010 issue of *Life Extension Magazine®*, the results of the largest study on 25-hydroxyvitamin D blood levels in dietary supplement users were published. These findings showed that most aging people require a dose of 5,000 IU and higher of supplemental vitamin D to attain optimal blood readings, which are now considered to be over 50 ng/mL.

References

1. http://www.taxpolicycenter.org/taxfacts/displayafact.cfm?Docid=407.
2. http://online.wsj.com/article/SB121556119847437537.html.
3. http://online.wsj.com/article/SB121556116413437535.html.
4. http://www.ustreas.gov/offices/public-affairs/hsa/pdf/pl108–173.pdf.
5. *Life Extension®*. 2007 Aug; 13(8):7–9.

6. http://www.miamiherald.com/428/v-print/story/628288. html.

7. *Rev Urol*. 2003;5 Suppl 5:S12–21.

8. *Urology*. 2009 May; 73(5):935–9; discussion 939.

9. *Prostate*. 2009 Jun 1; 69(8):895–907.

10. http://energycommerce.house.gov/Press_110/110nr383. shtml.

11. *Am J Clin Nutr*. 2008 Apr; 87(4):1080S–6S.

12. *Drugs Aging*. 2007; 24(12):1017–29.

13. *J Nutr*. 2005 Nov; 135(11):2739S–48S.

14. *QJM*. 1996 Aug; 89(8):579–89.

15. *Life Extension*. 2007 Oct; 13(10): 7–17.

16. *Am J Clin Nutr*. 2006 Jul; 84(1):18–28.

17. *J Nutr*. 2005 Nov; 135(11):2739S–48S.

18. *Med J Aust*. 2002 Aug 5; 177(3):149–52.

19. *Mayo Clin Proc*. 2003 Dec; 78(12):1457–9.

20. *N Engl J Med*. 2009 Apr 30; 360(18):1912–4.

21. *Crit Care Med*. 2004 Jun; 32(6):1254–9.

22. http://www.cms.hhs.gov/NationalHealthExpendData/02_ NationalHealthAccountsHistorical.asp.

23. http://www.cancer.org/docroot/PED/content/PED_10_2X_ Cigarette_Smoking_and_Cancer.asp

The Generic Drug Rip-off

I DID EVERYTHING I COULD—including risking life in prison. Back in the 1980s–1990s, the Life Extension Foundation® crusaded to enlighten Americans about the economic ruination that would occur if this country's corrupt drug regulatory structure was not abolished. At the behest of pharmaceutical interests, the FDA brutally retaliated against us.

What I am about to divulge is a shocking revelation about why prescription drugs cost so much. Before I describe this pervasive fraud, I want to remind readers what happens when an apathetic public allows archaic government regulations to rule the marketplace.

THE ECONOMIC COLLAPSE OF ARGENTINA

In the 1940s, Argentina was the ninth wealthiest country in the world. At one point it was richer than France and boasted a higher standard of living than Canada. It was considered one of the best countries in which to live.[1]

After an endless series of reckless governmental actions including uncontrolled borrowing and economic mismanagement, Argentina's standard of living ranking has plummeted to 46th.[2] If you had money in an Argentinean bank in 1999, it vanished. If you owned Argentinean government bonds, you lost most of your principal as the central government defaulted on its obligations.

Other countries have faced worse problems, including the mass murder of their citizens in one form or another by the central government.

The reason I mention Argentina is that its economic collapse has similarities to what the United States is facing. Misguided and corrupt government policies, combined with citizen apathy, allowed financial ruination to happen in Argentina. We in the United States are not immune to the same calamity.

If what I expose in this article does not motivate citizens to take action, I don't know what will. It is beyond my comprehension that the common-sense free market solution I propose will be ignored by the American citizenry.

HEALTHCARE COSTS BANKRUPTING UNITED STATES

Everything Life Extension® predicted about the healthcare cost crisis is happening before our eyes. Major corporations, individuals, and the government are being bankrupted by out-of-control medical costs. Some say the economic challenges facing the United States will result in substantially reduced standards of living. This does not have to happen.

As we long ago identified, the cause behind spiraling medical costs is a crooked and ludicrous regulatory structure.

Today's healthcare cost crisis is widely acknowledged and feared. No one, however, has yet proposed a practical solution to resolve it.

OVERPRICED DRUGS

The reason for high-priced generics is not because the active ingredients are expensive. On the contrary, compared with complicated nutrient extracts, the ingredients in drugs are usually synthetic chemicals that cost only pennies a day.

The culprit behind overpriced generic drugs is an archaic regulatory environment that functions to protect pharmaceutical financial interests, forcing consumers to pay artificially inflated prices for their generic medications.

If our proposal to overhaul today's inefficient regulatory system succeeds, at least part of the healthcare cost crisis will disappear quickly. A side benefit to lower-priced generic drugs is that it will force pharmaceutical companies to bring out life-saving medications faster, since almost-as-good generics will cost virtually nothing.

AN EXAMPLE OF A GROSSLY INFLATED GENERIC PRICE

Once a brand drug comes off patent, generic equivalents emerge, but they cost far more than they need to because of FDA overregulation.

Take the drug finasteride (Proscar®) for example. It came off patent in 2006, but at the end of 2008, chain pharmacies were charging about $90 for 30 tablets (a one-month supply). All it takes to make this drug is to put 5 mg of finasteride into a tablet that dissolves in the stomach. Vitamin companies do this every day with nutrients, but the FDA does not allow them to freely do the same thing with drugs.

We checked on the cost of buying finasteride and making it into tablets. The free market price for 30 tablets is only $10.25, which includes an independent assay of the ingredient quality, potency, and tablet dissolution—and a reasonable profit margin. It is against the law, however, for GMP-certified (Good Manufacturing Practices) vitamin manufacturers to offer low-cost generic drugs. This prohibition must be lifted as America can no longer afford to subsidize those who are politically connected while the country is driven into insolvency.

Finasteride is a drug that not only helps relieve benign prostate enlargement, but may also reduce the risk of prostate cancer.[3-5] Widespread use could save Medicare lots of money in expensive prostate treatments.

As evidence mounts about the prostate cancer risk reduction associated with drugs like finasteride, more companies are competing to make it, but its average price at chain pharmacies is around $86 a month—a staggering eight times higher than what its free market price would be!

Please note that generic prices tend to wildly fluctuate. In this case, as more competitors entered the market, chain pharmacies did not substantially lower the price of finasteride. In some cases, the opposite occurs, and by the time you read this, the price could vary.

HOW THE "GENERIC" REGULATORY SYSTEM WORKS

If a company wants to manufacture a generic drug, be it a prescription drug like finasteride or an over-the-counter (OTC) drug like ibuprofen, it must file an Abbreviated New Drug Application (ANDA) with the FDA, even if it is manufactured by others already.

While the company does not have to perform clinical trials for an ANDA, it does have to show its bioequivalence to the original drug. For drugs that are difficult to synthesize, this requirement is important. For most drugs, however, the raw material can be purchased, often from the identical supplier that provides it for the branded drug.

To show bioequivalence, the company typically needs to perform human studies that take 1.5–2 years, unless a sufficient number have already been performed successfully, in which case it might be able to use those prior studies to support the ANDA. But the FDA could reject the ANDA and require the company to perform studies anyway.

The cost and time involved in the ANDA process varies, depending on the drug, its safety, how long it has been on the market, etc.

To have an ANDA approved, it typically requires an investment of about $2 million, and it takes a total of two to three years to get the drug to market.

To manufacture a common drug like ibuprofen (the active ingredient in Advil® and numerous other OTCs) might cost about $1 million and take 1.5 years, because the company would not have to do its own studies, and because it is a drug with a known safety profile.

In addition to these costs, a company should budget 15% for legal fees, because wherever there is a big manufacturer with a sizable market share involved, they will sue, just to try to eliminate more competition from the market.

One's political connections with the FDA are critically important. Those who are not in the FDA's good graces might find it more difficult to get an ANDA approved. The company should have experience with this bureaucratic process to know when and how to object to unreasonable FDA requirements.

So as you can see, what should be a straightforward process to manufacture drugs like finasteride instead turns into a bureaucratic quagmire that results in generic drugs costing far more than they need to. If a person was to take 5 mg finasteride tablets made by a vitamin manufacturer, all they would need to do to document its efficacy would be to test their blood levels of dihydrotestosterone (DHT). Finasteride alleviates benign prostate enlargement symptoms by inhibiting the 5-alpha-reductase enzyme that converts testosterone into DHT. Properly made finasteride will lower DHT.

Under a free market system, consumers would have the choice of paying $86 for a one-month supply of FDA-approved generic finasteride, or $10.25 for a one-month supply of generic finasteride made by a GMP-certified (Good Manufacturing Practices)vitamin manufacturer.

HOW MUCH ARE YOU OVERPAYING?

Life Extension® investigators have spent an enormous amount of time identifying what it really costs to make a generic drug. The price of the active ingredient for most drugs is remarkably low. A greater expense involves GMP manufacturing and the kinds of quality control measures that we at Life Extension® mandate for the supplements that carry our label.

The chart opposite reveals the shocking numbers. Compared with what chain pharmacies are charging today, the free market prices are an astounding 51% to 94% lower!

On average, Americans are paying 837% more at chain pharmacies compared with what the free market price would be for the identical medications.

When looking at the ultra-low free market prices, it becomes evidently clear that there is no real prescription drug cost crisis. A month's supply of some of the most commonly used drugs could be obtained for the price of a box of cereal.

There never was a need for Congress to pass the thoroughly corrupt Medicare Prescription Drug Act that involves the massive expenditure of tax dollars to pay full retail prices for these hyper-inflated drugs.

GENERIC DRUG COMPARISON CHART

Brand Name	Generic Name	Average Price at Chain Drugstores	Free Market Price
Proscar®	Finasteride 5 mg	$ 86	$ 10.25
Zocor®	Simvastatin 20 mg	$ 27.99	$ 3.20
Norvasc®	Amlodipine 10 mg	$ 39.99	$ 4.41
Depakote®	Divalproex 500 mg	$ 129.99	$ 9.59
Lopressor®	Metoprolol 50 mg	$ 12.99	$ 2.21
Trileptal®	Oxcarbazepine 300 mg	$ 109.99	$ 15.50
Pravachol®	Pravastatin 40 mg	$ 51.99	$ 6.68
Altace®	Ramipril 10 mg	$ 61.99	$ 4.25
Lamictal®	Lamotrigine 100 mg	$ 119.99	$ 7.50
Neurontin®	Gabapentin 400 mg	$ 54.99	$ 5.85
Lotensin®	Benazepril 20 mg	$ 31.99	$ 4.40
Wellbutrin SR®	Bupropion 150 mg	$ 49.99	$ 17.99
Pamelor®	Nortriptyline 50 mg	$ 36.99	$ 4.39
Sonata®	Zaleplon 10 mg	$ 61.99	$ 12.43
Prilosec®	Omeprazole 20 mg (Rx)	$ 25.99	$ 12.70

The Free Market Prices listed on this chart are based on what an efficiently run pharmacy could sell these non-FDA-approved generics for. These prices would be lower if non-pharmacies were allowed to sell them. There are many expensive bureaucratic regulations that pharmacies have to adhere to, and the price of any drug you buy reflects the costs of complying with over-regulation of pharmacies, as well as over-regulation of generic drug manufacturing. The Free Market Prices on this chart would drop even further if large quantities of these non-FDA-approved generics were manufactured.

The free market price of generics would be so low, in fact, that even those with medical insurance will save money on most drugs compared with what their co-pays are now.

If these free market medications became available, medical insurance premiums will be lowered, Medicare's day of insolvency postponed, and many businesses and consumers spared from bankruptcy.

DOUBLE-DIGIT DRUG PRICE INCREASES SO FAR IN 2009

Despite inflation remaining at near zero this year, pharmaceutical companies are jacking up the prices they charge for patented drugs to even more exorbitant levels.

Since the Medicare Prescription Drug Act[6] requires the federal government to pay full retail price, pharmaceutical companies can literally name their price and receive guaranteed payment courtesy of taxpayers. Drug companies receive a substantial percentage of the retail price from private health insurers also, so the more they raise the prices, the more money they make.

Consumers are the ultimate victims. They face higher Medicare premiums and taxes, higher private insurance premiums, more exclusions and higher co-pays, and higher taxes to cover the $600 billion Medicare Prescription Drug Act.

Proposed legislation calls for the FDA to get more funding, so taxpayers may also be contributing to the bureaucracy that serves to protect drug companies against lower-priced competition.

The growing number of Americans without medical insurance and who don't qualify for government aid are priced out of the market for patented medications unless they are economically well-endowed. The federal government recognizes this problem and is proposing that even more tax dollars now be used to subsidize prescription drugs, though not at full retail price.

In fact, one reason pharmaceutical companies are increasing prices is that they fear the federal government will soon require they "discount" their patented medications. So the more they jack up the prices now, the greater amount they will receive after they are forced to lower them via government-mandated "discounts."

The chart below shows the double-digit price increases that occurred on popular drugs in the beginning of 2009.

RISING DRUG COSTS
Price of selected drugs, and change from previous year

Drug	Disease Treated	Dosage	Price (1Q 2009)	% change
Sprycel®	Leukemia	60 20-mg pills	$ 3,763.98	32.7%
Viagra®	Erectile dysfunction	30 25-mg pills	$ 519.46	20.7%
Strattera®	ADHD	30 10-mg pills	$ 159.28	15.6%
Sutent®	Kidney cancer	28 25-mg pills	$ 4,997.81	14.3%
Cialis®	Erectile dysfunction	30 20-mg pills	$ 551.17	14.2%

Source: Credit Suisse analysis based on Wolters, Kluwer, Price, Rx Pricing Database. This chart is reproduced from the Wall Street Journal, April 15, 2009. Reprinted with permission.

HOW CONSUMERS WILL BE PROTECTED

We are proposing that the law be amended to allow GMP-certified manufacturing facilities to produce generic prescription drugs that do not undergo the excessive regulatory hurdles that force consumers to pay egregiously inflated prices.

To alert consumers when they are getting a generic whose manufacturing is not as heavily regulated as it is currently, the law should mandate that the label of these less-regulated generic drugs clearly states:

This is not an FDA-approved manufactured generic drug and may be ineffective and potentially dangerous. This drug is NOT manufactured under the same standards required for an FDA-approved generic drug. Purchase this drug at your own risk.

By allowing the sale of these less costly generics, consumers will have a choice as to what companies they choose to trust.

The inevitable concern raised by this free market solution is safety. Who will protect consumers from poorly made generic drugs?

First of all, there will be the same regulation of these drugs as there are with GMP-certified supplement makers. FDA inspectors will visit facilities, take sample products, and assay to ensure potency of active ingredient, dissolution, etc. Laboratories that fail to make products that meet label claims would face civil and criminal penalties from the government.

Secondly, there is no incentive not to provide the full potency of active ingredient in these less-regulated generic drugs. The price of the active ingredients makes up such a small percentage of the overall cost that a manufacturer would be idiotic to scrimp on potency.

Companies that foolishly make inferior generics will be viciously exposed by the media, along with the FDA, consumer protection groups, and even prescribing physicians who will be suspicious if a drug was not working as it is supposed to.

Companies producing inferior products will be quickly driven from the marketplace as consumers who choose to purchase these lower-cost generics will seek out laboratories that have reputations for making flawless products.

These substandard companies would not only be castigated in the public's eye, but face civil litigation from customers who bought the defective generics. When one considers that GMP-certified manufacturing plants can cost hundreds of millions to set up, a company would be committing suicide if it failed to consistently produce generic drugs that at least met minimum standards.

THE SECRET ABOUT COMPOUNDING PHARMACIES
THE FDA DOES NOT WANT YOU TO KNOW!

If you're like most people, you think prescription drugs are only made by pharmaceutical companies. This myth causes Americans to pay outrageous prices for drugs that can be bought for a fraction of the price from compounding pharmacies.

For example, the price of a particular drug made by a major pharmaceutical company is $245 a month. You can obtain the identical quantity of this natural substance from a compounding pharmacy for as low as $29 a month! Since many insurance companies do not reimburse for this item, you would save over $2,592 a year by purchasing the compounded version of this drug as opposed one made by a pharmaceutical company. By law, I am not even allowed to mention the name of this drug. How's that for press freedom!

Pharmaceutical companies would prefer that you don't find out how to obtain your prescription drugs for 92% less than what you may now pay. That's why pharmaceutical giants lobby the FDA to incite the agency to censor compounding pharmacy advertising.

In a landmark legal case, the US Supreme Court ruled that the FDA violates the First Amendment's free speech provisions when it seeks to restrict advertising or promotion of compounded drugs. As a result of this Constitutional victory, you are now allowed to at least find out that there are compounded prescription medications available at a fraction of the price you have been paying. In fact, the cost for some compounded drugs is lower than co-pays for pharmaceutical company-manufactured ones.

MOLLIFYING THE CYNICS

No matter how many facts I list showing that these free market drugs will be safe, there are alarmists who believe that even if one person suffers a serious adverse event because of a defective generic drug, then the law should not be amended to allow the sale of these less-regulated products.

What few understand is that enabling lower-cost drugs to be sold might reduce the number of poorly made drugs. The reason is that prescription drug counterfeiting is a major issue today. Drugs are counterfeited because they are so expensive. With a month's supply of free market simvastatin selling for only $3.20, it is difficult to imagine anyone profiting by counterfeiting it. So amending the law to enable these super-low-cost drugs to be sold might reduce the counterfeiting that exists right now.

Another reason these less-regulated generics will do far more good than harm is that people who need them to live will be able to afford them. The media has reported on heart-wrenching stories of destitute people who cannot afford even generic prescription drugs. They either do without, or take a less-than-optimal dose. The availability of these free market generics will enable virtually anyone to be able to afford their medications.

PRESERVING OUR COUNTRY'S FINANCIAL FUTURE

The cost of prescription drugs is a significant factor in today's healthcare cost crisis, a problem that threatens to bankrupt consumers and this nation's medical system. Passage of common-sense legislation would quickly slash the cost of generic drugs so low that consumers could obtain them for less than what their co-pays currently are. Enormous amounts of money would be saved by public and private insurance programs, and ultimately consumers.

According to the Government Accountability Office (GAO), all federal revenue will be eaten up by government outlays for Medicare, Medicaid, Social Security, and public debt interest by 2025[7]—just 16 years from now!

We as a nation can no longer afford to be bound by today's inefficient regulatory system that artificially inflates the cost of our prescription medications. The money is no longer there to support this bureaucratic morass.

UPDATE

Those who think generic drugs are safe today should be aware of isolated instances when improperly made active ingredients make it into prescription drugs sold in US pharmacies. These defective ingredients often emanate from FDA-approved manufacturers in China and India. The FDA gives false assurances that these government-approved laboratories are safe. The reality is that the FDA can only inspect each Chinese drug making factory at best only once every 13 years[8]. So the protection consumers think they have today is a façade. I would feel more comfortable buying generics from a company that had its own inspectors in offshore manufacturing facilities as opposed to relying on meaningless FDA rhetoric.

References

1. www.wikipedia.org/wiki/Argentina.
2. www.hdrstats.undp.org/en/2008/countries/country_fact_sheets/cty_fs_ARG.html.
3. *Rev Urol.* 2003;5(Suppl 5):S12–21.
4. *Urology.* 2009 May;73(5):935–9; discussion 939.
5. *Prostate.* 2009 Jun 1;69(8):895–907.
6. www.citizen.org/congress/reform/rx_benefits/drug_benefit/.
7. www.house.gov/budget_republicans/entitlement/roadmap_detailed_entirereport.pdf.
8. "Beware the Risks of Generic Drugs," *Wall Street Journal*, July 6, 2011.

Ending the Atrocities

TODAY'S POPULATION LIVES on a railroad track. Everything may be fine for the moment—until a freight train comes along and wipes us out.

We at Life Extension® have pled for 29 years to get off the track before the train comes.

A startling number of reports reveal the FDA is in far worse shape than originally thought. Few people comprehend that they are likely to suffer and die prematurely as a result of FDA's failures.

The media does a decent job reporting on FDA disasters. The apathetic public, however, often forgets what they read the next day. That is, until they are diagnosed with a serious illness. Then they go into a panic mode to find an effective treatment. All too often, however, the cure does not exist because of FDA bureaucratic roadblocks. In other cases, the FDA-approved drugs available induce horrific side effects.

It is our mission to memorialize these tragedies to demonstrate the urgent need to radically reform the FDA. This "state-sponsored" carnage of the American citizenry must be stopped!

FDA DISSEMINATES FRAUDULENT SAFETY DATA

Ketek® is a drug the FDA approved to treat mild to moderate pneumonia. Ketek® can also cause sudden and serious liver damage. In some cases complete liver failure develops necessitating the need for a liver transplant. Some patients die before a liver transplant can be performed.[1]

The risks of liver failure (and other toxic side effects) were known *before* the FDA approved Ketek®. In order to convince an outside scientific advisory committee to recommend that Ketek® be approved, the FDA knowingly allowed a *fraudulent* safety study to be presented. Here is what the Senate Investigative Committee uncovered:[2]

- FDA accepted the resubmission of a new drug application that included safety data that was fraudulent, in whole or in part.
- FDA instructed its employees preparing to appear before the advisory committee that they should present this fraudulent safety data.
- FDA employees presented the fraudulent study data to the advisory committee tasked with recommending Ketek®'s approval or disapproval.
- FDA approved a pediatric clinical trial of Ketek®, involving infants as young as six months old, despite concerns related to known toxicities affecting the heart, eyes, liver and vascular system.
- FDA continued to knowingly cite the fraudulent study data in publically released safety information on Ketek®.

How fraudulent was this data? While the FDA was presenting this fake data, a criminal investigation was simultaneously being conducted that found the clinic where the "safety" study allegedly occurred was *closed* during the time the study was supposed to have taken place. It was also determined that documents relating to the safety study had date modifications and signature inconsistencies.

Shortly after the advisory committee meeting where the fake safety data was presented by FDA employees, the person who conducted the study was criminally indicted, pled guilty, and sentenced to almost five years in jail.

It is even more shocking that the FDA continued to cite this safety study long after the principal investigator admitted it was fraudulent. While the perpetrator of this "safety" study was in prison for falsifying the data, the FDA used the very same study to issue a Public Health Announcement stating:

> Based on the pre-marketing clinical data it appeared that the risk of liver injury with telithromycin (Ketek®) was similar to that of other marketed antibiotics.[3]

The "pre-marketing clinical data" FDA cited to tell the public that Ketek® was safe was the fraudulent study, a study that may never have actually occurred. According to the Senate Investigative Committee report, "it defies explanation why the FDA would continue to cite" this fraudulent study to the American public to imply that Ketek® is safe.[3]

The Senate Committee report concluded by stating that

> Retaliation against these individuals, or any other FDA employees who communicate with the committee with reference to Ketek® will not be tolerated.[4]

Based on the tone of the Senate investigative report, it would appear that the FDA functioned as a continuous criminal enterprise in this instance.[5, 6]

THE REVOLVING DOOR

You may wonder why certain officials in the FDA would go to such extreme lengths to get a lethal drug like Ketek® approved.

Look no further than the gargantuan economic benefits drug companies reap when a patented compound like Ketek® receives the FDA seal of approval.

When we first exposed the revolving door of FDA employees going to work for companies they regulate, virtually no one believed us. Back in the 1980s, most Americans were deceived by FDA propaganda stating that the agency "is responsible for protecting the public health by assuring the safety ... of human drugs."[9]

The harsh reality is that the FDA functions primarily to protect the financial interests of the pharmaceutical industry, not the public's health. If anyone ever questioned this, look no further than the FDA's attempts last year to ban the safest form of estrogen (estriol). The FDA has no qualms about publically stating their ban on estriol was based on a petition filed by Wyeth, the maker of dangerous estrogen drugs like Premarin® and PremPro®.

There are a number of estrogen drugs that have not been shown to increase stroke and breast cancer risk.[10] The FDA, however, has done nothing to remove Premarin® or Prem-Pro®. Instead, the FDA openly seeks to protect Wyeth's market share by denying American women access to natural estriol.

According to the FDA, "bioidentical hormone products are unsupported by medical evidence and are considered false and misleading by the agency."[11] The truth is that bioidentical hormones are far less expensive and pose a major competitive threat to Wyeth, ergo the FDA's aggressive attempts to disallow them.

In a report issued by the Associated Press just last year, it was revealed that a record number of FDA employees are leaving the agency to go to work for pharmaceutical companies. According to the Associated Press, these FDA staffers are resigning in order to go into "the more lucrative side of the business."[12]

THE FDA'S BRAIN DRAIN

As experienced FDA scientists leave the agency to work for Big Pharma, the remaining staff is leaner and less competent to approve new lifesaving medications. As reported by the Associated Press, a consequence of FDA employees going to work for pharmaceutical companies is a clogging of the drug approval pipeline.

As long time Life Extension® members know, the FDA drug approval process has always been a bureaucratic quagmire, where lifesaving medications languish for years, decades and sometimes forever. The drug pipeline has been "clogged" for almost 50 years. We are deeply disturbed that it is now taking even longer for lifesaving medications to become available to those in need.

The *Wall Street Journal* continues to support our position with blistering exposes on human beings who suffer horrendously and die while potential lifesaving therapies languish in the FDA approval process. An article published last year titled "Sick Patients Need Cutting-Edge Drugs," disclosed heart-wrenching reports of young cancer patients who were denied compassionate-use access to experimental drugs. The *Wall Street Journal* article raised the logical questions:

> Why do terminally ill patients have to wait so long to get access to the only treatments that hold any promise of saving their lives? And why is it not their right to decide?[13]

These very issues have been discussed in Life Extension's publications for nearly 30 years. We have analogized in previous articles how it is perfectly legal to engage in all kinds of risky activities, such as parachuting off of high bridges, but it is *illegal* to make experimental medications available to terminally ill people without the FDA's permission.

According to the *Wall Street Journal*, the drug delay problem is getting much worse. The problem has been magnified in recent years as the number of new drug approvals has fallen dramatically. The FDA approved just 16 new drugs in 2007 and only 17 in 2008.[14,15] That's down from 53 in 1996 and 39 in 1997.

With the approval of lifesaving drugs grinding to a snail's pace, the moronic cruelty of denying experimental drugs to terminal patients must stop. Each day a life saving drug is delayed, human beings perish. The case for radical reform of the Food, Drug, and Cosmetic Act and the FDA itself has never been stronger.

FDA BUNGLES NEW SYSTEM TO TRACK SIDE EFFECTS

Even when data used to approve a new drug is *not* fraudulent, there are inherent limitations in assessing toxic side effects in the clinical study setting. Reasons for this include the relatively short time period the drugs are evaluated in a clinical study compared to how long patients use them in the real world. Another problem is that clinical studies are often tightly controlled by doctors with specialized expertise in the particular drug they are evaluating. Practicing physicians, on the other hand, see dozens of patients a day and may not be familiar with the proper way to prescribe drugs that have a narrow safety window. Still another issue is the relatively small number of patients taking the drugs in a clinical study compared to the millions who may eventually be prescribed it.

Due to these serious limitations, post-approval surveillance is critical to identifying lethal side effects of prescription drugs that were not detected in the clinical trials.

According to a report by an independent auditing institute, the FDA squandered $25 million on a bungled computer system to track side effects of approved drugs.[16, 17] As a result, the FDA will have to rely on a dysfunctional system to track what are record breaking numbers of adverse reports being made about drugs the agency previously approved as safe.

After this report showing that FDA errors and mismanagement caused this system to not be available, the FDA asked that most of the findings of the report be deleted. The independent institute who put the report together refused to capitulate to the FDA's attempts to obstruct the report's findings.[17, 18]

DRUG PRICES SURGE

In today's upside down regulatory system, Americans are prescribed drugs whose approval may be based on fraudulent or insufficient research data. Experimental therapies that could save their lives are routinely denied. The *cost* of existing medications meanwhile is skyrocketing.

Drug price increases often exceed the inflation rate. The average increase for the top 50 best selling drugs was 7.82% in 2007, 6.73% in 2006, and 6.22% in 2005.[19]

Some very popular drugs are increasing at astronomical rates. The antidepressant Wellbutrin XL® went up by 44.5% from 2005 to 2007. The attention-deficit drug Adderall XR® went up by 33.5%. The price of the sleep-aid drug Ambien® shot up 70.1% during this period.[19]

On less popular drugs, the price surges are worse than obscene. A drug used to treat heart problems in premature babies went from $136.10 to $1,875.00 in one year. A drug used to treat a certain cancer (Cosmegen®) increased from $16.79 to $593.75 in one year. A drug used to treat spasms in babies (Acthar) was increased from about $1,650.00 to more than $23,000.00 in one year. Just imagine your baby suffering spasms and being asked to fork over $23,000.00 for one drug![20]

DO DRUG COMPANIES HAVE *ANY* DECENCY?

It is beyond my comprehension to understand how pharmaceutical companies can look themselves in the mirror when they know they are selling drugs proven to kill.

Back in 1994, our best selling product was shark cartilage. The problem we uncovered was that it was not curing cancer patients. We immediately notified our customers that a survey we conducted of those who bought shark cartilage showed it to be ineffective. We urged these people to seek other therapies.

The supplement industry was shocked at our findings, but most stopped promoting shark cartilage as anti-cancer therapy. Our findings about shark cartilage's lack of efficacy were confirmed several years later in a controlled study.

We were a relatively small organization in 1994 and losing our best selling product was financially challenging. In no way, however, could we continue telling cancer patients that shark cartilage might help them when our own findings showed it did not work.

The fact the multibillion dollar pharmaceutical companies have no qualms about using fraudulent data to support the approval and continued sale of lethal drugs is an atrocity. That certain people within the FDA collude with pharmaceutical companies to allow dangerous and ineffective drugs on the market is an act so heinous that words do not exist to describe it.

Whether you use these drugs or not, you still suffer. The thoroughly corrupt Medicare Prescription Drug Act passed at the behest of pharmaceutical lobbyists mandates that taxpayers pay full retail prices for these drugs.[21] Taxpayers will fork over $600 billion for these egregiously overpriced drugs in the first ten years.[22]

Where consumers are really hurt is in their ever-increasing health insurance premiums. If you are fortunate enough to have someone else paying your premiums, you cannot help but note the higher deductibles and greater exclusions.

The FDA enables drug companies to financially rape the American consumer by stifling competition. There are so many regulatory hurdles to getting FDA approval for even a competitive generic drug that consumers often pay eight times more than they need to.

Under the guise of "consumer protection," the FDA has been manipulated by pharmaceutical interests to restrict free market forces that would drive down drug costs.

FDA BOTCHES PUBLIC RELATIONS CAMPAIGN

The FDA has been pummeled by Congress and the media about its many scandals, including poor inspections of tainted foods, drugs and other products it regulates.

Needless to say, this has created a severe image problem. So FDA officials decided to hire a public relations agency that would "create and foster a lasting positive public image of the agency for the American public," according to agency documents.[23]

When taxpayer dollars are involved, the law mandates a bidding process be used to ensure that the contract go to the lowest cost contractor. According to an exposé published by the *Washington Post*, the propaganda contract went instead to a public relations firm with ties to the FDA official who arranged the deal. A loophole was used to avoid putting the contract up for bid.[24]

After being made aware of this apparent corrupt act, an FDA deputy commissioner suspended the public relations contract and ordered an independent investigation.

Congress responded by launching still another investigation into the FDA. According to the chairman of the House committee that oversees the FDA, "The agency chose to use its limited resources to save face instead of saving the public health."[25]

The FDA retains the power to make life and death decisions that affect all of us. When it comes to analyzing new therapies to extend human longevity, this involves the scientific and common sense ability to understand complex biochemical interactions that occur within living organisms. The FDA's botched attempt to launch a misinformation campaign to cover up its inadequacies further calls into question its competency and moral legitimacy.

FIGHTING BACK

In 1994, we established the FDA Museum to document how the FDA's failings were responsible for the needless deaths of millions of Americans.

Sadly, every assertion we made about the FDA back then has been validated by third parties and the FDA itself. I lament that we were proven correct, because this means that millions more Americans perished unnecessarily over the past 15 years . . . and the cost of today's corrupt healthcare system threatens to financially decimate our country.

The FDA's credibility is at an all-time low. There has never been a better time to enact legislation to reform the way healthcare is regulated in this country. With a new Congress in session, health freedom activists are aggressively seeking to have the law changed to allow free market forces to tear down the corrupt wall of bureaucracy that causes the needless death of thousands of Americans each day.

HOW MANY DRUG-INDUCED SUICIDES?

The same Senate committee investigating the Ketek® scandal uncovered another study with falsified data. This fake data was used to support the approval of a popular antidepressant drug used by millions of human beings.

According to a report authored by a Harvard medical doctor, when the Paxil® application was submitted to an FDA advisory committee in 1991, the drug company improperly counted those taking the real drug as placebo subjects. This was done to make it appear there to be no difference in the risk of suicidal behavior in those taking Paxil® compared to placebo.

It took until year 2006 for the manufacturer to send a letter to doctors admitting the risk of suicidal behavior was 6.7 times higher in study subjects taking Paxil® as compared to placebo.[7]

Suicide is the 11th leading cause of death in the United States.[8] It killed over 34,000 people in year 2004. The number of suicides attributed to drugs like Paxil® (select serotonin reuptake inhibitors) could be in the hundreds of thousands during the 13 years it was fraudulently marketed.[4,5]

We at Life Extension® are working with the American Association for Health Freedom (AAHF)* to make our voices heard in Congress. AAHF is a coalition of integrative physicians, healthcare consumers, and health freedom activists committed to a complete reform of the FDA. Its Reform FDA Petition is available for signing at www.ReformFDA.org.

* AAHF is now the Alliance for Natural Health USA (ANH–USA). Their website is http://www.ANH-USA.org.

More scientific innovation is occurring in the medical field than at any time in human history. This progress is irrelevant, however, if a regulatory barrier denies the fruits of this research to people in need, or allows drugs to be sold with lethal side effects, or renders the cost of medications unaffordable.

The Life Extension Foundation® has been battling FDA ineptitude for three decades. Your support enables us to continue this ongoing struggle to convince Congress to radically reform the way healthcare is controlled in this country.

References

1. Available at: http://www.drug-injury.com/druginjurycom/2007/12/ketek-case-repo.html. Accessed December 5, 2008.

2. Available at: http://www.druginjuryblog.com/2008/06/11/ketek-fraudulent-clinical-trials-prove-fda-not-doing-its-job-congress-says/. Accessed December 5, 2008.

3. Available at: http://www.fda.gov/ora/about/enf_story2006_archive/ch3/default.pdf. Accessed December 5, 2008.

4. Available at: http://www.ketekliverinjury.com/liver_failure/study.html. Accessed December 5, 2008.

5. Available at: http://finance.senate.gov/press/Gpress/2007/prg122007a.pdf. Accessed December 5, 2008.

6. Available at: http://www.senate.gov/~finance/press/Gpress/2008/prg061208.pdf. Accessed December 5, 2008.

7. Available at: http://us.gsk.com/docs-pdf/media-news/Paxil-CR-and-Paxil-Adult-Suicide.pdf. Accessed December 5, 2008.

8. Available at: http://www.cdc.gov/ncipc/dvp/suicide/SuicideDataSheet.pdf. Accessed December 5, 2008.

9. Available at: http://www.fda.gov/opacom/morechoices/mission.html. Accessed December 5, 2008.

10. Available at: http://www.mayoclinic.com/health/breast-cancer/WO00092. Accessed December 5, 2008.

11. Available at: http://www.fda.gov/bbs/topics/NEWS/2008/ NEW01772.html. Accessed December 5, 2008.

12. Available at: http://www.msnbc.msn.com/id/24953413/ wid/7279844/. Accessed December 5, 2008

13. Available at: http://cei.org/articles/sick-patients-need-cutting-edge-drugs.

14. Available at: http://www.pharmacistsletter.com/pl/newdrugs/ FDA2007.pdf?cs=&s=PL. Accessed December 5, 2008.

15. Available at: http://pharmacytechniciansletter.com/pl/newdrugs/ FDA2008.pdf?cs=&s=PTL. Accessed December 5, 2008.

16. Available at: http://www.ahrp.org/cms/content/view/ 476/28/. Accessed December 5, 2008.

17. Available at: http://www.ahrp.org/cms/index2.php?option= com_content&do_pdf=1&id=476.

18. Available at: http://finance.senate.gov/press/Bpress/2007press/ prb030707a.pdf. Accessed December 5, 2008.

19. Available at: http://online.wsj.com/article/ SB120355185318681367.html. Accessed December 5, 2008.

20. Available at: http://assets.aarp.org/rgcenter/post-import/ dd113_generic_drugs.pdf. Accessed December 5, 2008.

21. Available at: http://www.ustreas.gov/offices/public-affairs/ hsa/pdf/pl108–173.pdf. Accessed December 5, 2008.

22. Available at: http://www.aafp.org/fpm/20050300/49what. html. Accessed December 5, 2008.

23. Available at: http://www.nytimes.com/2008/10/05/ opinion/ 05sun4.html?ref=opinion. Accessed December 5, 2008.

24. Available at: http://www.washingtonpost.com/wp-dyn/ content/article/2008/10/01/AR2008100103061_pf.html. Accessed December 5, 2008.

25. Available at: http://energycommerce.house.gov/ Press_110/110nr 362.shtml. Accessed December 5, 2008.

Millions of
Needless Deaths

T IS HARD TO IMAGINE, but it was not until 1867 that Joseph
Lister published his findings about the critical need of
using sterile procedures in the surgical setting. Back
then, doctors seldom washed their hands prior to surgery,
let alone sterilize the instruments they had used on the
previous patient.

Before Dr. Lister's sterile techniques were adopted,
patients frequently died from infections introduced during surgery.

Joseph Lister had little interest in financial or social
success. These traits enabled him to endure the criticisms
hurled by the medical establishment about the extra steps
he took to ensure his surgical environments were clean.

One of Dr. Lister's greatest challenges was to persuade his
colleagues that germs did in fact exist. Back then, most doctors still believed in the theory of spontaneous generation.[1]

Convincing today's medical establishment about proven methods to save lives may be less daunting than what Dr. Lister encountered, but it is still nonetheless challenging.

TODAY'S BODY COUNT

Back in 2007, I urged the federal government to declare a national emergency. My rationale was that millions of Americans were going to needlessly die if the epidemic of vitamin D insufficiency was not immediately corrected. My article was based on irrefutable scientific evidence documenting how vast numbers of lives could be spared if everyone took at least 1,000 IU of vitamin D3 each day.[2]

I went a step further and showed how mandatory vitamin D supplementation could resolve today's healthcare cost crisis by slashing the need for expensive prescription drugs and hospitalizations.[2]

I took it two steps further and offered to donate 50,000 one-year-supply bottles of vitamin D3 so the government could give these away to those who could not afford this ultra-low cost supplement.[2]

It is now 16 months later. The federal government has done nothing to inform the public of the opportunity to radically reduce their risk of dying by taking a supplement that costs less than six cents a day!

VITAMIN D MORE EFFECTIVE THAN PREVIOUSLY KNOWN

A large number of new vitamin D studies have appeared in the scientific literature since I wrote my plea to the federal government. These studies don't just confirm what we knew 16 months ago—they show that optimizing vitamin D intake will save even more lives than we projected.

For instance, a study published in June 2008 showed that men with low vitamin D levels suffer 2.42 times more heart attacks. Now look what this means in actual body counts.[3]

Each year, about 157,000 Americans die from coronary artery disease-related heart attacks.[4] Based on this most recent study, if every American optimized their vitamin D status, the number of deaths prevented from this kind of heart attack would be 92,500.

To put the number of lives saved in context, tens of millions of dollars are being spent to advertise that Lipitor® reduces heart attacks by 37%. This is certainly a decent number, but not when compared with how many lives could be saved by vitamin D. According to the latest study, men with the higher vitamin D levels had a 142% reduction in heart attacks.[3]

This does not mean that you should stop taking medications if you can't get your cardiac risk factors under control by natural methods. It does mean that you should make certain you are not vitamin D-insufficient.

Please note that all forms of heart disease kill over 869,700 Americans each year.[4] These lethal forms of heart disease include cardiomyopathy, valvular insufficiency, congestive heart failure, arrhythmia, coronary thrombosis (blood clot in coronary artery), and coronary atherosclerosis (narrowing or blockage of coronary arteries). There is reason to believe that vitamin D could help protect against most of these forms of cardiac-induced death.

BILLIONS OF DOLLARS IN HEALTHCARE SAVINGS

There are 920,000 heart attacks suffered in the United States every year.[4] According to the American Heart Association, the annual cost of healthcare services, medications, and lost productivity related to these heart attacks is over $156 billion.[4]

The annual retail cost of all 300 million Americans (including children) supplementing with 1,000 IU of vitamin D per day is $6.6 billion.

So if vitamin D's only benefit was to reduce coronary heart attack rates by 142%, the net savings (after deducting the cost of the vitamin D) if every American supplemented properly would be around $84 billion each year. That's enough to put a major dent in the healthcare cost crisis that is forecast to bankrupt Medicare and many private insurance plans.

SPARING COUNTLESS NUMBERS FROM THE AGONIES OF CANCER

The evidence supporting the role of vitamin D in preventing common forms of cancer is now overwhelming.[2]

Vitamin D-deficient women, for example, have a 253% increased risk of colon cancer.[6] Colon cancer strikes 145,000 Americans each year and 53,580 die from it.[7] Based on these studies, if everyone obtained enough vitamin D, 38,578 lives could be saved and medical costs would be reduced by $3.89 billion.[8,9]

A study published in January 2008 showed that women with the lowest level of vitamin D were at a 222% increased risk for developing breast cancer.[10] Most studies show that higher levels of vitamin D can reduce breast cancer incidence by around 30–50%.[11–14]

Each year, approximately 186,800 women are diagnosed with breast cancer and 40,950 perish from it in the United States.[15] This needless toll of suffering and death caused by insufficient intake of vitamin D is unconscionable.

Prostate cancer will be diagnosed in an estimated 189,000 American men this year. Almost 30,000 will die from it.[16] Some studies show that men with higher levels of vitamin D have a 52% reduced incidence of prostate cancer.[17]

The first-year costs of prostate cancer treatment are approximately $14,540.[18] If all aging men achieved sufficient vitamin D status, about $1.4 billion could be saved each year.

So as you can see, there is no real healthcare cost crisis. What the population suffers from is frighteningly low blood levels of vitamin D. During winter months in Canada, for instance, an estimated 97% of the population is vitamin D-deficient.[19]

VITAMIN D PROTECTS AGAINST STROKE

Stroke is the number three cause of death in the United States.[20] It is also one of the most feared diseases because of its high incidence of permanent disability.

In a study published in September 2008, blood indicators of vitamin D status were measured in 3,316 patients with suspected coronary artery disease. The subjects were followed for 7.75 years. For every small decrease in blood indicators of vitamin D status, there was a startling 86% increase in the number of fatal strokes.[21]

The doctors who conducted this study concluded:

> Low levels of 25(OH)D* and 1,25(OH)2D* are independently predictive for fatal strokes, suggesting that vitamin D supplementation is a promising approach in the prevention of strokes.[21]

If all that vitamin D did was to reduce stroke risk, it would be critically important for every American to ensure optimal blood levels.

---

* 25[OH]D and 1,25[OH]2D are blood markers that measure vitamin D status in one's body.

LOW VITAMIN D DOUBLES DEATH RATE

Vitamin D deficiency is a worldwide problem. Yet no conventional medical organization or governmental body has declared a health emergency to warn the public about the urgent need of achieving sufficient vitamin D blood levels.

According to John Jacob Cannell, MD, founder of the nonprofit Vitamin D Counsel:

> Current research indicates vitamin D deficiency plays a role in causing seventeen varieties of cancer as well as heart disease, stroke, hypertension, autoimmune diseases, diabetes, depression, chronic pain, osteoarthritis, osteoporosis, muscle weakness, muscle wasting, birth defects, and periodontal disease.

> This does not mean that vitamin D deficiency is the only cause of these diseases, or that you will not get them if you take vitamin D. What it does mean is that vitamin D, and the many ways in which it affects a person's health, can no longer be overlooked by the healthcare industry nor by individuals striving to achieve and maintain a greater state of health.[22]

Vitamin D seems to reduce the risk of almost every killer disease of aging. In fact, a recent study shows that humans with low vitamin D status are twice as likely to die over a seven-year time period![5]

Each year, the federal government spends $1 billion in research aimed at finding ways to prevent or cure the killer diseases of aging.[23] Yet the government is oblivious to the most medically effective and cost-effective way of preventing needless death. This is analogous to how the establishment ignored Joseph Lister's pleas for a sterile environment in the surgical arena.

DIFFERENCE BETWEEN "DEFICIENCY" AND "INSUFFICIENCY"

Doctors are not trained to recognize a vitamin D deficiency until rickets develop in children or osteomalacia (softening of the bones) develops in adults. Clinical vitamin D deficiency is diagnosed when blood levels of a vitamin D metabolite (25-hydroxyvitamin D) drop below 12 ng/mL.

According to the world's foremost experts, however, optimal blood levels of vitamin D are between 30 and 50 ng/mL and higher.[24,25] Those with blood levels below 30 ng/mL are considered to have insufficient vitamin D.

These widely varying numbers explain why mainstream medicine is at a loss to understand the widespread health problem created by less than optimal vitamin D levels. If physicians view a patient's medical chart and see a vitamin D blood level of 18 ng/mL, they will think this person has adequate vitamin D. The reality is that a vitamin D blood level this low predisposes this patient to virtually every killer disease of aging and may in fact be the reason that individual has become a "patient" instead of remaining healthy.

There clearly is a need for a new consensus in the medical community to redefine vitamin D deficiency as a blood reading below 30 ng/mL. As we at *Life Extension*® long ago learned, it can take decades for the establishment to change its reference ranges to reflect scientific reality.

WHAT CAN BE DONE?

Despite the startling number of needless deaths, the federal government has done nothing to warn the public of the lethal dangers associated with vitamin D insufficiency.

We will distribute my original 2007 article along with this editorial to every member of the new Congress and the President in January 2009. Hopefully someone will understand the urgency of declaring a health emergency and advise that every American maintain a vitamin D blood level of at least 30 ng/mL (and preferably above 50 ng/mL).

If the government continues to ignore our pleas, perhaps private insurance companies will consider sending free bottles of vitamin D supplements to all of their subscribers. The outlays for medical procedures and prescription drugs would be expected to plummet in groups who took their vitamin D supplement each day.

The media has done a good job in reporting on the numerous positive findings about vitamin D over the past two years. Sales of vitamin D supplements have been increasing, so at least some Americans are getting the message and taking steps to guard against vitamin D insufficiency.

In the meantime, *Life Extension®* will continue to report on new findings about vitamin D. We have found that if we repeat a message long enough, much of the public will wake up to scientific reality and the desire for self-preservation.

ALL HOSPITALIZED PATIENTS SHOULD BE TESTED FOR VITAMIN D

The pioneer of antiseptic procedures in the hospital setting was a Hungarian physician named Ignaz Semmelweis. In one of the world's great detective stories, Dr. Semmelweis went back 100 years to find out why there was such an increase in puerperal fever (childbed fever) that had killed thousands of mothers in obstetric units.

Dr. Semmelweis correlated increases in autopsies performed at hospitals with greater incidences of lethal puerperal fever. It turned out that doctors would leave an autopsy room with their hands covered in decomposing human tissues (and lots of bacteria) and deliver babies with their fetid hands.

Semmelweis instructed his interns to wash their hands with chlorinated lime solutions and documented an immediate reduction in puerperal fever incidence.

Despite the logic of his arguments and concrete proof shown by the reduction in mortality when handwashing procedures were followed, Semmelweis faced a wall of opposition. Back in those days, maternity hospitals had horrendous reputations and were sometimes referred to as deathtraps. Some suggested that lives could be saved simply by closing the clinics where people went in with minor problems and ended up dying agonizing deaths. Doctors of the day refused to accept that they were the ones responsible for the deaths of thousands of young women. Semmelweis was eventually committed to an insane asylum where he died.

Move forward to 2009, and hospitals are still places to avoid. Medical errors, antibiotic-resistant infections, sleep interruption, pneumonia, and malnutrition continue to ravage those confined to the hospital setting.

An overlooked problem with institutional confinement is that patients admitted with insufficient vitamin D can rapidly develop severe vitamin D deficiency due to complete lack of sunlight and malnutrition caused by commotion in the hospital environment.

A strong argument could be made that every patient admitted to a hospital should have their blood tested for vitamin D and supplements administered to ensure that blood levels remain considerably above 30 ng/mL. The improvement in immune function along with reduced inflammatory responses alone could result in many more patients leaving via the hospital lobby rather than its morgue.

There are respected medical authorities today advocating universal vitamin D supplementation, but their pleas are all but ignored by most practicing doctors. Unlike the plight of women in childbirth exposed to puerperal fever by ignorant doctors in the past, no informed person has to suffer from lack of vitamin D. More and more people are taking their supplements with them when they go to the hospital because they know they will need them there more than in any other place.

WHERE TO PURCHASE VITAMIN D

Fortunately, the patent for synthesizing vitamin D expired long ago. It is an ultra-low-cost supplement available at any health food store, pharmacy, and most grocery stores. There is no economic impediment precluding immediate widespread supplementation.

Please know that we remain relentless in tearing down the walls of medical ignorance that are by far the leading causes of disability and death in the United States.

IMPORTANT UPDATE

In 2009, the Life Extension Foundation® conducted the largest study ever on blood levels of vitamin D in dedicated dietary supplement users. The startling findings revealed that 85% of the study subjects had less than optimal vitamin D blood levels, defined as having 25-hydroxyvitamin D below 50 ng/ml. Based on these unexpected findings, aging humans were encouraged to increase their supplemental vitamin D intake to between 5,000 IU and 10,000 IU each day. A full report on this study can be found in the January 2010 issue of *Life Extension Magazine*® located at www.lef.org.

References

1. Available at: http://en.wikipedia.org/wiki/Abiogenesis. Accessed September 4, 2008.

2. Faloon W. Should the president declare a national emergency? *Life Extension.* 2007 Oct;13(10):7–17.

3. Giovannucci E, Liu Y, Hollis BW, Rimm EB. 25-hydroxyvitamin D and risk of myocardial infarction in men: a prospective study. *Arch Intern Med.* 2008 Jun 9;168(11):1174–80.

4. Available at: www.americanheart.org/downloadable/ heart/1200082005246HS_Stats%202008.final.pdf. Accessed October 29, 2008.

5. Dobnig H, Pilz S, Scharnagl H, et al. Independent association of low serum 25-hydroxyvitamin d and 1,25-dihydroxyvitamin d levels with all-cause and cardiovascular mortality. *Arch Intern Med.* 2008 Jun 23;168(12):1340–9.

6. Holick MF. Vitamin D and sunlight: strategies for cancer prevention and other health benefits. *Clin J Am Soc Nephrol.* 2008 Sep;3(5):1548–54.

7. Available at: www.cdc.gov/cancer/colorectal/statistics/. Accessed September 4, 2008.

8. Lappe JM, Travers-Gustafson D, Davies KM, Recker RR, Heaney RP. Vitamin D and calcium supplementation reduces cancer risk: results of a randomized trial. *Am J Clin Nutr.* 2007 Jun;85(6):1586–91.

9. Brown ML, Lipscomb J, Snyder C. The burden of illness and cancer: economic cost and quality of life. *Annu Rev Public Health.* 2001;22:91–113.

10. Abbas S, Linseisen J, Slanger T, et al. Serum 25-hydroxyvitamin D and risk of post-menopausal breast cancer—results of a large case-control study. *Carcinogenesis.* 2008 Jan;29(1):93–9.

11. Rossi M, McLaughlin JK, Lagiou P, et al. Vitamin D intake and breast cancer risk: a case-control study in Italy. *Ann Oncol.* 2008 Aug 18.

12. Giovannucci E. Vitamin D and cancer incidence in the Harvard Cohorts. *Ann Epidemiol.* 2008 Feb 19.

13. Abbas S, Linseisen J, Chang-Claude J. Dietary vitamin D and calcium intake and premenopausal breast cancer risk in a German case-control study. *Nutr Cancer.* 2007;59(1):54–61.

14. Robien K, Cutler GJ, Lazovich D. Vitamin D intake and breast cancer risk in postmenopausal women: the Iowa Women's Health Study. *Cancer Causes Control.* 2007 Sep;18(7):775–82.

15. Available at: www.cdc.gov/cancer/breast/statistics/. Accessed October 28, 2008.

16. Available at: www.cdc.gov/cancer/prostate/statistics/. Accessed October 28, 2008.

17. Li H, Stampfer MJ, Hollis JB, et al. A prospective study of plasma vitamin D metabolites, vitamin D receptor polymorphisms, and prostate cancer. *PLoS Med.* 2007 Mar;4(3):e103.

18. Wilson LS, Tesoro R, Elkin EP, et al. Cumulative cost pattern comparison of prostate cancer treatments. *Cancer.* 2007 Feb 1;109(3):518–27.

19. Available at: http://vitamins-minerals.suite101.com/article.cfm/the_sunshine_vitamin; http://www.vitamindsociety.org/. Accessed September 4, 2008.

20. Available at: www.cdc.gov/nchs/fastats/deaths.htm. Accessed September 4, 2008.

21. Pilz S, Dobnig H, Fischer JE, et al. Low vitamin D levels predict stroke in patients referred to coronary angiography. *Stroke.* 2008 Sep;39(9):2611–3.

22. Available at: http://74.125.45.104/search?q=cache:fgZo6Q5-SO8J:www.vitamindcouncil.org /+Current+research+indicates+vitamin+D+deficiency+plays+a+role+in+causing+seventeen& hl=en&ct= clnk&cd=1&gl=us. Accessed September 4, 2008.

23. Available at: www.nia.nih.gov/AboutNIA/NACA/MeetingInformation/DirStatusReportMay2007.htm. Accessed September 4, 2008.

24. Vieth R. Vitamin D supplementation, 25-hydroxyvitamin D concentrations, and safety. *Am J Clin Nutr.* 1999 May;69(5):842–56.

25. Holick MF. The role of vitamin D for bone health and fracture prevention. *Curr Osteoporos Rep.* 2006 Sep;4(3):96–102.

2008

Would You Tolerate This Abuse?

AMERICANS NEEDLESSLY DIE while scientific discoveries that could save their lives remain trapped in bureaucratic red tape.

There is a solution to this travesty. Allow free market innovation into the healthcare arena, and the development of new medical therapies will progress as rapidly as other technologies.

Do you remember how expensive long distance phone calling used to be?

Back in 1980, archaic federal rules enabled the original AT&T to control national long distance dialing. You could recognize a long distance call by the hissing and crackling noise heard before the caller spoke. High-speed Internet and mobile phone connections were not available.

CONSUMERS FOUGHT BACK

There was quite a debate around 1980 as to whether consumers would benefit if other companies were allowed to compete in offering long distance services. AT&T heavily lobbied Congress arguing that all kinds of terrible problems would occur if it lost its monopoly.

AT&T pointed to its stellar record of scientific advances and threatened that if it could not charge its monopolistic rates, then further improvements in communications technology would be hindered. AT&T's track record for scientific prowess gave them a strong argument.

Fortunately, free market theory prevailed and AT&T was forced to relinquish its stranglehold over long distance calling in the United States. The transition was by no means smooth. The initial long distance competitors' services were clearly inferior to AT&T. One newspaper columnist complained that he was tired of being solicited by these substandard discount carriers and wanted the government to reinstate AT&T's monopoly.

HOW TIMES HAVE CHANGED

Anyone who has paid attention to long distance rates over the past 28 years appreciates the enormity of the benefit brought about by abolishing AT&T's monopoly.

Consumers used to pay over 60 cents per minute for daytime long distance calls (equal to $1.39 per minute in today's depreciated dollars).[1] Can you imagine if you had to pay $250 for three hours of long distance calling? This would be unthinkable today where for under $40 a month, you can have an unlimited long distance service that usually includes local connection charges.

Consumers today save a whopping 84% compared with 1980, even if they only make three hours of long distance calls a month. Unlike AT&T's threats of technological stagnation, the quality, reliability, and speed of today's long distance phone service are vastly superior.

WHY DO AMERICANS TOLERATE PHARMACEUTICAL MONOPOLIES?

What if the federal government outlawed long distance competition and returned to the monopolistic ways of the past? If this were to occur, every elected politician who voted for this would be thrown out of office.

Yet the public today tolerates federal and state laws that enable pharmaceutical companies to conduct business as a virtual monopoly. The result is that Americans pay outlandish prices for mediocre drugs that are often laden with side effects.

As AT&T did in 1980, drug companies seek to deceive Congress and the public by stating their high prices are needed in order to discover better technologies. The reality is that after decades of exorbitant drug pricing, one's odds of surviving a serious disease using conventional methods are not substantially improving. Yet drug prices are exponentially higher.

Citizen apathy has allowed this economic and medical bloodbath to occur. One of Life Extension's missions is to provide the hard facts so that today's antiquated regulatory system can be eradicated. We believe that in a free market environment, technological breakthroughs that occurred in telecommunications will also happen in medicine.

UNREGULATED SUPPLEMENT PRICES PLUMMET

Unlike regulated prescription drugs, the cost of dietary supplements has plummeted over the past three decades.

For example, when coenzyme Q10 (CoQ10) was first introduced to Americans in 1983, a bottle containing 1,000 mg (100 10-mg capsules) retailed for $30. In 2008, the retail price of a bottle containing 5,000 mg (100 50-mg capsules) of a superior form of CoQ10 (ubiquinol) is $58.

Based on milligram potency alone, the cost in inflation-adjusted dollars for CoQ10 has come down by 83%.

If the FDA had succeeded in turning CoQ10 into a drug as it tried to do in the early 1980s, you might be paying $337.50 for what retails now for $58.

Under the FDA's regulatory stranglehold, it is unlikely that the superior ubiquinol form of CoQ10 would have been "approved" any time soon. This would force Americans to pay the inflated price ($337.50 per bottle) for a less-than-optimal product. This illogic is what monopolies are all about, and why they cannot be allowed to exist.

If one looks at the price history of dietary supplements, costs are substantially lower now than when they were originally brought out. When SAMe was first introduced to Americans in 1996, it cost $45 for 4,000 mg (twenty 200 mg tablets). This was the European-regulated "drug" price. Soon after it became an *unregulated* supplement, the price went down a great deal. As more manufacturers competed to make SAMe, the price plummeted to where Life Extension® members can obtain 8,000 mg (twenty 400 mg tablets) for only $21. Thus SAMe now costs 77% less than when it was originally introduced.

Prescription drug costs, on the other hand, have skyrocketed at a rate that far exceeds inflation. The difference is that prescription drugs are heavily regulated, as opposed to dietary supplements that are sold under free market conditions.

TODAY'S HEALTHCARE CATASTROPHE

Today's healthcare calamities are so numerous it is not possible to fit them into one issue of *Life Extension Magazine®*. To remind you of news reports published in 2008, we reprinted a few of the appalling headlines at the end of this chapter.[2–10]

As you can clearly see by these reports, unless radical legal changes are made, Americans will continue to pay high prices for dangerous drugs that have limited efficacy.

More frightening is the suffocating effect that regulation has on the discovery of life-saving therapies. Just imagine if advancement in clinical medicine progressed at the same rapid rate as telecommunications. If it did, we would probably have cures for most killer diseases today!

For example, the first direct-dial transcontinental telephone call occurred in 1951.[11] That first call took 18 seconds to complete, had lots of static in the background, and most consumers could not readily afford it. Move forward to 2008, and we all have access to clear phone connections across the country instantly at minimal cost.

Now look at the dire prognosis for pancreatic cancer patients today. A patient diagnosed with pancreatic cancer in 2008 typically lives just a few months longer compared with 1951.[12–14] Yet the price for these additional months of life can be thousands of times higher than that in 1951.[15]

We need to swiftly improve medical science at a speed analogous to telecommunications, computers, and other unregulated technologies.

SCATHING FDA REPORT PROVIDES BASIS TO REVOLUTIONIZE MEDICINE

The FDA has provided a rare opportunity to enact legislation that can enable Americans to quickly gain access to life-saving medical therapies.

The FDA recently did a study of itself and its findings revealed that it is scientifically incompetent and incapable of doing its job.[16,17] These are not mere allegations from outside critics, but are instead the FDA itself admitting that it cannot carry out its mission.

There has never been a better time for a comprehensive overhaul of the FDA. Everything about it—from its mission to its management—needs to be taken apart, reviewed, redefined, and recreated so that it helps support, rather than obstruct, a vibrant free market in healthcare science.

CAN LOGIC PREVAIL OVER LETHAL DOGMA?

There are pessimists who think Americans will not be able to achieve true health freedom in the immediate future. Naysayers complain that if free market principles are extended to healthcare, some terminally ill patients will die sooner if experimental therapies fail.

Again, review what happened when long distance phone calling was deregulated. Sure, there were problems in the beginning, but look at where we are today with a dependable low-cost phone service affordable to all. Even more impressive are the incredible advancements in high-speed internet access and mobile phone connectivity that would have been unthinkable in the early 1980s.

Life Extension's enthusiasm for a free market approach to healthcare is based on its confidence in judging which novel medical therapies are truly safe and effective. A look at *Life Extension's* 28-year track record shows that it has been able to identify life-saving approaches to combating disease long before they are approved by the FDA.

Has LEF made mistakes? Yes, we have fallen victim to a few fraudulent studies that caused us to recommend products that we later found did not work. We have not, however, recommended products that killed anyone. Contrast this to regulated FDA-approved drugs that have collectively killed millions of Americans over the past three decades.

The logic of letting the free market determine what therapies Americans may use to prevent and treat disease will defeat the cynics who fear changing the regulatory quagmire that exists today. Existing laws that protect against real health fraud will still enable charlatans to be stopped and prosecuted.

HEADLINE NEWS QUOTES FROM 2008 FORESHADOW TODAY'S HEALTHCARE CRISIS

THE $34 TRILLION PROBLEM

Medicare is poised to wreak havoc on the economy. And our politicians are avoiding the issue.[2]

ELI LILLY SETTLES ZYPREXA® LAWSUIT

$15 million settlement announced; state of Alaska alleged the drug caused health problems that cost Medicaid program hundreds of millions.[3]

STUDY: DRUG ERRORS HURT ONE IN FIFTEEN HOSPITALIZED KIDS

Medicine errors, overdoses, bad reactions harm one in 15 hospitalized kids. This estimate translates to 7.3% of hospitalized children, or 540,000 kids annually. Patient safety experts say that the problem is most likely even bigger than the study suggests.[4]

US LAGS BEHIND FORTY-ONE NATIONS IN LIFE SPAN

For decades, the United States has been slipping in international rankings of life expectancy, as other countries improve healthcare, nutrition, and lifestyles.[5]

FDA BLAMED FOR DIP IN NEW DRUGS

New drug approvals down 31% so far this year: report; FDA still stinging from Vioxx® approval.[6]

BUREAUCRATIC OBSTACLES SHOULDN'T STAND IN THE WAY OF THE TERMINALLY ILL

Back in 2001, a vivacious, 21-year-old student at the University of Virginia—Abigail Burroughs—died of cancer. Her death was particularly heart-wrenching because, in the final weeks of her life, she was denied access to two investigational anti-cancer drugs recommended by her oncologist. The FDA later approved the drugs.[7]

US REPORTS OF DEATH, SIDE EFFECTS FROM PRESCRIPTION DRUGS TRIPLE

Reports of dangerous side effects and deaths from widely used medicines almost tripled between 1998 and 2005, an analysis of US drug data found.[8]

WOMAN LEFT IN CT SCANNER AFTER CLINIC CLOSES

A cancer patient says she was left alone in a CT scanner for hours after a technician apparently forgot about her. She finally crawled out of the device, only to find herself locked in the closed clinic. Doctor says it has happened before.[9]

BREAST CANCER PATIENTS MAY FACE MORE HEART RISK

Breast cancer survivors may face increased risk of heart disease. Doctors are debating if it is time to largely abandon a chemotherapy mainstay that is one reason for the problem.[10]

References

1. *Consumer Reports*. 1983. Nov;48(11): 618–20.
2. Available at: http://money.cnn.com/2008/03/03/news/economy/104239768.fortune/index.htm. Accessed June 23, 2008.
3. Available at: http://www.newsinferno.com/archives/1589. Accessed June 23, 2008.
4. Available at: http://www.cnn.com/2008/HEALTH/04/07/children.drug.errors.ap/index.html. Accessed June 23, 2008.
5. Available at: http://www.boston.com/news/education/higher/articles/2007/08/11/us_life_span_shorter/. Accessed June 23, 2008.
6. Available at: http://money.cnn.com/2007/08/15/news/companies/fda/index.htm. Accessed June 23, 2008.

7. Available at: http://blogs.usatoday.com/oped/2007/08/ our-view-on-exp.html. Accessed June 23, 2008.

8. Available at: http://www.foxnews.com/story/0,2933,296427, 00.html. Accessed June 23, 2008.

9. Available at: http://www.msnbc.msn.com/id/21033714/. Accessed June 23, 2008.

10. Available at:http://www.kmov.com/justposted/stories/ kmov_health_071008_breastcancerheart.14e95c1d0.html. Accessed June 23, 2008.

11. Available at: http://www.corp.att.com/attlabs/reputation/ timeline/51trans.html. Accessed June 23, 2008.

12. Stewart RJ, Stewart AW, Stewart JM, Ibister WH. Cancer of the pancreas in New Zealand 1970–1974. *Aust N Z J Surg.* 1982 Aug;52(4):379–84.

13. Available at: http://www.pancreatica.org/Pancreatica%20 Media%20Sheet.pdf. Accessed June 26, 2008.

14. Czernichow P, Lerebours E, Colin R. *Epidemiology* of cancer of the pancreas. Current data. *Presse Med.* 1986 Feb 22;15 (8):387–91.

15. Available at: http://www.medscape.com/viewarticle/409001_2. Accessed June 26, 2008. 16 Faloon W. The FDA indicts itself. *Life Extension.* 2008 July;14(7):7–11.

16. Available at: http://www.fda.gov/ohrms/dockets/AC/07/ briefing/2007-4329b_02_01_FDA%20Report%20on%20 Science%20and%20Technology.pdf. Accessed June 23, 2008.

17. Available at: http://www.apma.net/aahf/default.asp. Accessed June 23, 2008.

The FDA Indicts Itself

BACK IN THE EARLY 1980S, Life Extension® predicted horrific tragedies if government control over healthcare was not abolished. The heartbreaking fact is that tens of millions of Americans have needlessly suffered and died because of FDA incompetence . . . and the FDA now admits its own incompetence!

These tens of millions of lives lost are not statistics of strangers. Virtually everyone has family or friends who have been victimized by dangerous drugs or denied access to life-saving ones.

FDA UNCOVERS ITS OWN INADEQUACIES

The FDA, in collusion with pharmaceutical giants and conventional medical orthodoxy, is the leading cause of suffering and death in the United States.

Back in the early days, the FDA would defend its position by proclaiming that it served to protect the public's health. An endless number of well-publicized scandals have caused the FDA itself to admit that it is incapable of carrying out its mission.[1–10]

If all the FDA did was act so cautiously that it almost never approved a dangerous drug, then at least the agency could point to some consumer value it provides. Instead, we are plagued by an antiquated regulatory agency that stifles the development of novel life-saving medications, while allowing a slew of drugs to be sold that have cumulatively cost millions of lives.

Americans thus suffer the "worst of both worlds" as they are poisoned by FDA-sanctioned prescription drugs, but denied the fruits of novel approaches to disease prevention and treatment.

FDA'S INDICTMENT OF ITSELF

In response to a barrage of criticisms, FDA commissioner Dr. Edward von Eschenbach requested that a special committee assess whether the FDA is capable of doing its job. The premise for the FDA's massive audit of itself was the fear that "the nation is at risk if FDA science is at risk."

Their sixty-page report, entitled "FDA Science and Mission at Risk,"[11] states that "the world of drug discovery and development has undergone revolutionary change," but the FDA's "evaluation methods have remained largely unchanged over the last half century. "

The following are exact quotes from the report:

- The FDA cannot fulfill its mission because its scientific base has eroded and its scientific organizational structure is weak.
- The FDA cannot fulfill its mission because its scientific work force does not have sufficient capacity and capability.

- The FDA cannot fulfill its mission because its information technology (IT) infrastructure is inadequate.
- The FDA does not have the capacity to ensure the safety of food for the nation.
- The development of medical products based on "new science" cannot be adequately regulated by the FDA.
- There is insufficient capacity in modeling, risk assessment, and analysis.
- The FDA science agenda lacks a coherent structure and vision, as well as effective coordination and prioritization.
- The FDA has substantial recruitment and retention challenges.
- The FDA has an inadequate and ineffective program for scientist performance.
- The FDA has not taken sufficient advantage of external and internal collaborations.
- The FDA lacks the information science capability and information infrastructure to fulfill its regulatory mandate.
- The FDA cannot provide the information infrastructure support to regulate products based on new science.

Most appalling is the FDA's own finding that it "cannot even keep up with the advances in science."[11] Said differently, this means that the FDA cannot keep up with scientific breakthroughs that could cumulatively save millions of human lives!

RESPONSES TO THE FDA'S DAMNING REPORT OF ITSELF

The *Wall Street Journal* wrote an editorial titled "The Real FDA Scandal" and quoted the following about the FDA's admitted statement:

Particularly in complex and specialized fields like genomics and biotechnology medicine, the FDA lacks the basic competence "to understand the impact of product use, to maintain ongoing currency with their evolution or to evaluate the sophisticated products produced" and "to support innovation in the industries and markets that it regulates."[12]

The *Wall Street Journal* further wrote, "Think about that: We live amid a revolution in biology, but the FDA still thinks like it did when Sputnik launched."[12]

Dr. David Kessler was the most publicly recognized FDA commissioner of all time. Dr. Kessler is still sought out by the media as a proponent on FDA issues. In response to this horrific report, however, Dr. Kessler stated, "The problems are way bigger than one commissioner. . . . I'm not sure how anybody could do this job now."[13]

FDA commissioner Eschenbach stated, "I think to do what we need to do requires substantially more dollars than what has been invested in the FDA so far. . . . This is a systemic overhaul that must go on for years."[13]

PROBLEMS ARE WORSE THAN FDA ADMITS

Many recent reports from outside organizations have been harshly critical of the FDA. These reports made national news for a day or two and were then quickly forgotten.[14-24]

Our greatest impediment to saving human lives is an incompetent and corrupt federal bureaucracy that is strangling medical innovation, especially in the areas of genomics and biotechnology where breakthroughs in anti-aging medicine are most expected.

In discussions with scientists about methods to significantly extend our life spans, the problem with "the FDA" inevitably arises. If the FDA's bureaucratic roadblock is not torn down, we may all succumb to a disease that liberated scientists could readily prevent or cure.

There is not a magic immortality pill that the FDA is directly suppressing. Instead, the FDA is restraining the ability for medical science to progress. This is no longer just opinion. The FDA itself admits it cannot keep up with advances in science. So discoveries that could save human lives are not getting approved by the FDA and the cost is thousands of American lives being lost each day.

WHAT CAN BE DONE TO STOP THIS CARNAGE

There are a number of proposals to turn around this lethal barrier to medical progress called the Food and Drug Administration (FDA). Some politicians say throw more tax dollars at the problem, while other politicians refuse to reward an agency with so much documented incompetence.

The FDA's own report makes it clear that scientific innovation is suffocated by bureaucratic red tape and incompetency. Yet a medical renaissance is needed if our generation is to achieve dramatically extended life spans.

The only way to liberate scientific ingenuity is to allow Americans to obtain therapies that are clearly marked "Not approved by the FDA." Under this free market scenario, those who want the so-called "protection" the FDA previously pretended it provided could continue receiving it.

Enlightened individuals and their doctors, on the other hand, would be able to choose novel therapies that are clearly labeled "Not approved by the FDA."

Since it costs so much for a new drug to be approved, therapies that do not have to go through this arduous (and antiquated) approval process would cost less than outlandishly priced "approved" prescription drugs.

DON'T LET MEDICAL INNOVATION BE HELD HOSTAGE TO FDA BUREAUCRACY!

Back in 2003, *Life Extension*® initiated a poll on a website that has about 400,000 new visitors each month.[25] The people visiting this site are not part of any anti-FDA group, nor were they exposed to anti-FDA teachings. These people were asked a simple question as to whether terminally ill cancer patients should have the right to any drug that might save their life. The results, after 22,506 votes were tabulated:

TERMINALLY ILL CANCER PATIENTS:

- Should have access to any drug that might save their life: **89%**
- Should only have access to drugs approved by the FDA: **11%**

We live in a constitutional republic where the people's wishes are supposed to be adhered to (so long as they don't infringe on the rights of others). If 89% of the American public thinks terminal cancer patients should have access to any drug that could save their life, then there is no reason for the law not to be changed to allow Americans to access therapies "Not approved by the FDA."

Companies that engage in fraud could be prosecuted under consumer protection laws that already exist. The FDA could post its opinion about the safety and efficacy of unapproved therapies on its website (www.fda.gov). The civil litigation risks to companies that knowingly sell bogus products would preclude large-scale unsavory activities that some are concerned with. The greater fear Americans face is being diagnosed with a lethal disease only to find out that a cure is nowhere in sight.

REACTIONS TO THE FDA'S CONFESSION

The FDA's admission that it cannot do its job has stirred up a hornet's nest of outrage from organizations who have long argued that the FDA is the greatest impediment to the advancement of medical science.

A new bill has been drafted that is being presented by health freedom activists to our friends in Congress. Passage of this bill into law will liberate Americans from the FDA's nearly 50-year tyrannical rule over what therapies an individual is allowed to choose to remain alive. A remarkable number of divergent health organizations are finally recognizing the lethal consequences of ignoring the FDA's ineptitudes and have committed to backing this legislation.

American citizens deserve the right to choose what goes into their bodies. Those who prefer therapies that are "Not approved by the FDA" should be allowed to do so, especially now that the FDA has come to the conclusion that it is too incapable and incompetent to keep up with scientific advances.

UPDATE

Regrettably, the Congressional bill that would have given terminal patients access to experimental therapies was not enacted into law. Pharmaceutical giants represent a huge special interest that does not want innovative nimble companies competing to bring out better therapies at lower prices. Big Pharma enjoys record profits by selling antiquated therapies at outlandish prices and lobbies hard to protect its sordid quasi-monopoly.

References

1. Available at: http://www.naturalnews.com/002157.html. Accessed March 19, 2008.

2. Available at: http://www.drugresearcher.com/news/ng. asp?id=58116-fda-in-the. Accessed March 19, 2008.

3. Available at: http://www.drugresearcher.com/news/ ng.asp?id=60304-whistleblowers-reveal-fda. Accessed March 19, 2008.

4. Available at: http://www.lawyersandsettlements.com/ articles/00680/ketek-scandal.html. Accessed March 19, 2008.

5. Available at: http://www.mises.org/story/1805. Accessed March 19, 2008. Accessed March 19, 2008.

6. Available at: http://www.ghchealth.com/the-aspartame-scandal.html. Accessed March 19, 2008.

7. Available at: http://healthcarescandals.wordpress.com/ category/fda/. Accessed March 19, 2008.

8. Available at: http://www.twnside.org.sg/title2/health.info/ twninfohealth034.htm. Accessed March 19, 2008.

9. Available at: http://www.naturalnews.com/002439.html. Accessed March 19, 2008.

10. Available at: http://query.nytimes.com/gst/fullpage.html?r es=950DE4DD1E38F930A2575BC0A96F948260. Accessed March 19, 2008.

11. Available at: http://www.fda.gov/ohrms/dockets/AC/07/ briefing/2007-4329b_02_01_FDA%20Report%20on%20 Science% 20and%20Technology.pdf. Accessed March 20, 2008.

12. Available at: http://online.wsj.com/article/SB120225742208745 785.html?mod=opinion_main_review_and_outlooks. Accessed March 20, 2008.

13. Available at: http://online.wsj.com/article/SB1204075529255 95245.html?mod=distsmartbrief&apl=y&r=49040. Accessed March 20, 2008.

14. Available at: http://money.cnn.com/2007/08/15/news/ companies/fda/index.htm. Accessed March 21, 2008.

15. Available at: http://www.safecosmetics.org/your_health/index.cfm. Accessed March 21, 2008.

16. Available at: http://www.cspinet.org/foodsafety/. Accessed March 21, 2008

17. Available at: http://goliath.ecnext.com/coms2/gi_0199-5599197/GAO-report-criticizes-FDA-drug.html. Accessed March 21, 2008.

18. Available at: http://ahrp.blogspot.com/2008/03/gao-to-investigate-fda-review-process.html. Accessed March 21, 2008

19. Available at: http://www.newsinferno.com/archives/2585. Accessed March 21, 2008.

20. Available at: http://www.ahrp.org/cms/content/view/46/28/. Accessed March 21, 2008.

21. Available at: http://www.uspirg.org/uspirg.asp?id2=24595. Accessed March 21, 2008.

22. Available at: http://www.iom.edu/CMS/3793/26341/37329.aspx. Accessed March 21, 2008.

23. Available at: http://www.lifesitenews.com/ldn/2006/aug/06082405.html. Accessed March 21, 2008.

24. Available at: http://www.psrast.org/bghsalmonella.htm. Accessed March 21, 2008.

25. Available at: www.deathclock.com. Accessed March 21, 2008.

The FDA's Cruel Hoax

D O YOU REMEMBER HOW POPULAR tryptophan was in the 1980s? Back in those days, people seeking to lose weight, improve sleep, or alleviate depression used tryptophan to safely increase serotonin levels in their brain.

Serotonin is the natural compound that promotes feelings of wellbeing, satiety, and relaxation. A serotonin deficiency can result in sleep disturbance, anxiety, depression, and a propensity to overeat.

In 1989, the FDA restricted the importation of tryptophan. This forced American consumers to switch to expensive prescription drugs that produced only partial effects at best.

Tryptophan is an amino acid found naturally in the foods that we eat. The reason its sale was stopped was because of defective tryptophan made by a substandard company.

The FDA's prejudicial position against tryptophan caused Americans to suffer widespread deficiencies of serotonin in their brains. A result of serotonin deficiency may be reflected in today's epidemic of obesity, depression, anxiety, and insomnia.

TRYPTOPHAN IS BACK!

Despite intense lobbying efforts by pharmaceutical companies, the FDA could not rationally continue to block the sale of tryptophan. After all, tryptophan is not only found in food, but the very tryptophan that the FDA restricted is still used in infant formulas and intravenous feeding solutions. If there were any danger to tryptophan, we would have known about it long ago.

Pharmaceutical-pure tryptophan can now be imported for use in dietary supplements. This means that aging Americans may be able to discard certain prescription drugs and once again treat their serotonin deficiency disorder with what Mother Nature intended all along . . . the amino acid tryptophan itself!

A FINANCIAL WINDFALL FOR THE DRUG COMPANIES

At the time that the FDA restricted tryptophan, it was the most popular dietary supplements sold in the United States. Perhaps it is a coincidence, but since 1989, the percentages of overweight and obese adult Americans have soared. Could it be that a nationwide serotonin deficiency has led to the high-carbohydrate overeating syndrome that so many Americans suffer from today?

The removal of tryptophan created an economic windfall for the drug companies. Sales of drugs that interfere with the brain's reuptake of serotonin (like Prozac®, and later Paxil® and Zoloft®) shot through the roof, earning tens of billions of dollars of profits for drug companies. While these drugs caused large numbers of unpleasant and possibly lethal side effects, the FDA withdrew none of them.

The ensuing epidemic of weight gain and sleeplessness resulted in dozens of anti-obesity and anti-insomnia drugs being approved by the FDA, some of which had horrendous side effects, and others that had virtually no efficacy.

Critics contend that the contaminated tryptophan coming from one substandard Japanese company provided a convenient excuse for the FDA to restrict the sale of all tryptophan dietary supplements. The FDA's actions guaranteed that Americans would become tryptophan-deficient, and therefore turn to prescription drugs for relief from a host of disorders related to insufficient serotonin in the brain.

PHARMACEUTICAL-PURE TRYPTOPHAN NOW AVAILABLE

Consumers now have access to pharmaceutical-pure tryptophan as an over-the-counter dietary supplement. According to the FDA, it is now the responsibility of the company who sells the tryptophan to ensure that it is not contaminated.

For 19 years, aging Americans have been forced to settle for less-than-optimal levels of tryptophan/serotonin in their bodies.

Based on what has been published in the peer-reviewed scientific literature, it would appear that consumers have suffered enormously from a host of disorders related to lack of serotonin in the brain.

Pharmaceutical companies, on the other hand, have accumulated exorbitant wealth, as depressed, overweight, and sleep-deprived consumers were forced to experiment with costly and side effect-laden drugs in order to combat the effects of serotonin deficiency.

If tryptophan dietary supplements provide relief to those suffering from common age-related disorders such as anxiety, depressed mood, sleeplessness, and unwanted weight gain, the FDA's nearly two-decade restriction on this natural agent may turn out to be one of the cruelest hoaxes of all time.

2006

Fish Oil Now Available by Prescription!

OR DECADES, THE PHARMACEUTICAL INDUSTRY has sought to limit competition by trying to get the FDA to regulate high-potency supplements as drugs. It was only because of intense consumer backlash that Congress passed legislation that protected the free sale of most supplements in the United States.

The introduction of an overpriced prescription fish oil drug provides absolute proof that every letter to Congress was well worth sending. Americans were perceptive enough to not let the drug industry (and federal government) trample our liberties under the guise of "protecting" us against "unproven" products.

PRESCRIPTION FISH OIL

The scientific evidence documenting the effects of fish oil in the body is overwhelming.[1-3] One of the substantiated benefits of fish oil supplementation is lowering elevated triglycerides in the blood.[4-6]

An enterprising company used the scientific findings about fish oil and conducted a study on humans with extremely high triglycerides (over 500 mg/dL).[7] As would be expected, compared to placebo, the triglyceride levels of the patients who received the fish oil were reduced by 51.6%. This company then applied to the FDA to have its fish oil approved as a new drug. The FDA granted the approval based on the company-sponsored clinical study showing that fish oil does exactly what it had previously been shown to do—that is, lower triglyceride levels.

With prescription drug status, this company is now free to make specific health claims about fish oil and aggressively sell it through cardiologists. If this company's marketing efforts are successful, it stands to earn an enormous amount of money from unwitting patients who do not realize that they can obtain fish oil supplements for a fraction of the price of this prescription fish oil drug.

WHY WOULD YOU EVER BUY YOUR FISH OIL BY PRESCRIPTION?

This new prescription fish oil product, containing 180 one thousand-milligram capsules per bottle, costs a whopping $236.89! That is about nine times more expensive than what this amount of fish oil sells for in a health food store.

The company selling this prescription fish oil drug knew that some consumers might question why they should pay such a high price. In their marketing materials, the company tries to differentiate their fish oil drug from what is available in health food stores by stating the following:

The US Food and Drug Administration (FDA) has not approved nonprescription, dietary supplement omega-3s for the treatment of any specific disease or medical condition, like very high triglyceride levels. Dietary supplement omega-3, or so-called fish oil, is not a substitute for prescription (fish oil) because they are not bioequivalent.[8]

Those who feel more comfortable using FDA-approved products can choose to pay the outlandish price of $236.89 for each bottle of this prescription-only fish oil drug. Even people with health insurance may find that their co-pay for this fish oil drug is still higher than what they could freely pay for fish oil supplements at a health food store. That is to say nothing of how much health insurance premiums could increase if too many patients are deceived into using this overpriced fish oil drug.

GREATER CONCENTRATION OF EPA/DHA IN PRESCRIPTION FISH OIL

This expensive fish oil drug does provide more EPA and DHA in each capsule than do most fish oil products sold by supplement companies. What this means is that five or six ordinary fish oil capsules might be needed to get the same amount of EPA/DHA contained in four capsules of this prescription-only version. But on a cost-per-milligram basis, the price for the prescription fish oil is still much higher than the non-prescription supplement.

WHAT OTHER NEW PRESCRIPTION FISH OIL DRUGS MIGHT THE FDA APPROVE?

Fish oil has been shown to prevent or alleviate a wide variety of ailments, including depression,[9-19] osteoporosis,[20-23] arthritis,[24-28] stroke,[29-31] heart attack,[32-44] Alzheimer's disease,[45-54] and some forms of cancer.[55-61]

Might there be future prescription fish oil products approved by the FDA as antidepressant drugs, as bone-protecting prescription drugs, as anti-arthritis prescription drugs, and even as cancer-preventive prescription drugs?

If so, some drug companies stand to make a lot of money. Elderly patients who are unaware of lower-cost fish oil supplements might have to do without some basic necessities in order to afford their fish oil prescriptions. This is unfortunate, as these high-priced fish oil drugs provide the same omega-3 fatty acids that health-conscious Americans have been supplementing with for the past 35 years.

UPDATE

Perhaps in response to harsh criticism, the price of prescription drug fish oil has dropped somewhat since its introduction in 2006, but it is still exponentially higher priced than what can be found in health food stores.

References

1. Guesnet P, Alessandri JM, Vancassel S, Zamaria N. Analysis of the 2nd symposium "Anomalies of fatty acids, ageing and degenerating pathologies." *Reprod Nutr Dev*. 2004 May–Jun;44(3):263–71.

2. Horrocks LA, Yeo YK. Health benefits of docosahexaenoic acid (DHA). *Pharmacol Res*. 1999 Sep;40(3):21 1–25.

3. Roland I, De Leval X, Evrard B, Pirotte B, Dogne JM, Delattre L. Modulation of the arachidonic cascade with omega3 fatty acids or analogues: potential therapeutic benefits. *Mini Rev Med Chem*. 2004 Aug;4(6):659–68.

4. Available at: http://www.ahrq.gov/news/press/pr2004/omega3pr.htm. Accessed June 29, 2006.

5. Bruckner G. Microcirculation, vitamin E and omega 3 fatty acids: an overview. *Adv Exp Med Biol*. 1997; 415:195–208.

6. Mori TA, Vandongen R, Beilin LJ, Burke V, Morris J, Ritchie J. Effects of varying dietary fat, fish, and fish oils on blood lipids in a randomized controlled trial in men at risk of heart disease. *Am J Clin Nutr*. 1994 May;59(5):1060–8.

7. Harris WS, Ginsberg HN, Arunakul N, et al. Safety and efficacy of Omacor in severe hypertriglyceridemia. *J Cardiovasc Risk*. 1997 Oct-Dec;4(5–6):385–91.

8. Available at: http://www.omacorrx.com/About_OMACOR/What_to_Expect_on_OMACOR.html. Accessed June 29, 2006.

9. Visioli F, Galli C. Oleuropein protects low density lipoprotein from oxidation. *Life Sci*. 1994;55(24):1965–71.

10. Tiemeier H, Van Tuijl HR, Hofman A, Kiliaan AJ, Breteler MM. Plasma fatty acid composition and depression are associated in the elderly: the Rotterdam Study. *Am J Clin Nutr*. 2003 Jul;78(1):40–6.

11. Su KP, Huang SY, Chiu CC, Shen WW. Omega-3 fatty acids in major depressive disorder. A preliminary double-blind, placebo-controlled trial. *Eur Neuropsychopharmacol*. 2003 Aug;13(4):267–71.

12. Nemets B, Stahl Z, Belmaker RH. Addition of omega-3 fatty acid to maintenance medication treatment for recurrent unipolar depressive disorder. *Am J Psychiatry*. 2002 Mar;159(3):477–9.

13. Peet M, Horrobin DF. A dose-ranging study of the effects of ethyl-eicosapentaenoate in patients with ongoing depression despite apparently adequate treatment with standard drugs. *Arch Gen Psychiatry*. 2002 Oct;59(10):913–9.

14. Edwards R, Peet M, Shay J, Horrobin D. Omega-3 polyunsaturated fatty acid levels in the diet and in red blood cell membranes of depressed patients. *J Affect Discord*. 1998 Mar;48(2–3):149–55.

15. Peet M, Murphy B, Shay J, Horrobin D. Depletion of omega-3 fatty acid levels in red blood cell membranes of depressive patients. *Biol Psychiatry*. 1998 Mar 1;43(5):315–9.

16. Maes M, Christophe A, Delanghe J, Altamura C, Neels H, Meltzer HY. Lowered omega-3 polyunsaturated fatty acids in serum phospholipids and cholesteryl esters of depressed patients. *Psychiatry Res*. 1999 Mar 22;85(3):275–91.

17. Stoll AL, Severus WE, Freeman MP, et al. Omega-3 fatty acids in bipolar disorder: a preliminary double-blind, placebo-contolled trial. *Arch Gen Psychiatry*. 1999 May;56(5):407–12.

18. Hibbeln JR. Fish consumption and major depression. *Lancet.* 1998 Apr 18;351(9110):1213.

19. Maes M, Smith R, Christophe A, et al. Fatty acid composition in major depression: decreased omega 3 fractions in cholesteryl esters and increased C20: 4 omega 6/C20:5 omega 3 ratio in cholesteryl esters and phospholipids. *J Affect Disord.* 1996; 38:35–46.

20. Kruger MC, Coetzer H, de Winter R, Gericke G, van Papendorp DH. Calcium, gamma-linolenic acid (GLA) and eicosapentaenoic acid (EPA) supplementation in senile osteoporosis. *Aging* (Milano). 1998 Oct;10(5):385–94.

21. van Papendorp DH, Coetzer H, Kruger MC. Biochemical profile of osteoporotic patients on essential fatty acid supplementation. *Nutr Res.* 1995; 1 5(3):325–34.

22. Bhattacharya A, Rahman M, Banu J, et al. Inhibition of osteoporosis in autoimmune disease prone MRL/Mpj-Fas(lpr) mice by N-3 fatty acids. *J Am Coll Nutr.* 2005 Jun; 24(3):200–9.

23. Kesavalu L, Vasudevan B, Raghu B, et al. Omega-3 fatty acid effect on alveolar bone loss in rats. *J Dent Res.* 2006 Jul;85 (7):648–52.

24. Berbert AA, Kondo CR, Almendra CL, Matsuo T, Dichi I. Supplementation of fish oil and olive oil in patients with rheumatoid arthritis. *Nutrition.* 2005 Feb;21 (2): 131–6.

25. de la Puerta R, Martinez-Dominguez E, Ruiz-Gutierrez V. Effect of minor components of virgin olive oil on topical antiinflammatory assays. *Z Naturforsch* [C]. 2000 Sep-Oct;55(9–10):814–9.

26. Alexander JW. Immunonutrition: the role of omega-3 fatty acids. *Nutr.* 1998 Jul-Aug;14(7–8):627–33.

27. Ariza-Ariza R, Mestanza-Peralta M, Cardiel MH. Omega-3 fatty acid in rheumatoid arthritis: an overview. *Semin Arthritis Rheum.* 1998 Jun;27(6):366–70.

28. Kremer JM, Lawrence DA, Petrillow GF, et al. Effects of high-dose fish oil on rheumatoid arthritis after stopping non-steroidal antiinflammatory drugs. *Arthritis Rheum.* 1995 Aug;38(8):1107–14.

29. Serhan CN. Novel eicosanoid and docosanoid mediators: resolvins, docosatrienes, and neuroprotectins. *Curr Opin Clin Nutr Metab Care*. 2005 Mar;8(2):1 15–21.

30. Li H, Ruan XZ, Powis SH, et al. EPA and DHA reduce LPS-induced inflammation responses in HK-2 cells: evidence for a PPAR-gamma-dependent mechanism. *Kidney Int*. 2005 Mar;67(3):867–74.

31. Iso H, Rexrode KM, Stampfer MJ, et al. Intake of fish and omega-3 fatty acids and risk of stroke in women. *JAMA*. 2001 Jan 1 7;285(3):304–1 2.

32. Thorngren M, Gustafson A. Effects of 11-week increases in dietary eicosapentaenoic acid on bleeding time, lipids, and platelet aggregation. *Lancet*. 1981 Nov 28;2(8257):1 190–3.

33. Hjerkinn EM, Seljeflot I, Ellingsen I, et al. Influence of long-term intervention with dietary counseling, long-chain n-3 fatty acid supplements, or both on circulating markers of endothelial activation in men with long-standing hyperlipidemia. *Am J Clin Nutr*. 2005 Mar;81 (3):583–9.

34. Trichopoulou A, Bania C, Trichopoulou D. Mediterranean diet and survival among patients with coronary heart disease in Greece. *Arch Intern Med*. 2005 Apr 25;165(8):929–35.

35. Mori TA, Beilin LJ. Omega-3 fatty acids and inflammation. *Curr Atheroscler Rep*. 2004 Nov;6(6):461–7.

36. Calder PC. n-3 fatty acids and cardiovascular disease: evidence explained and mechanisms explored. *Clin Sci* (Lond). 2004 Jul; 107(1): 1–11.

37. Yam D, Bott-Kanner G, Genin I, Shinitzky M, Klainman E. The effect of omega-3 fatty acids on risk factors for cardiovascular diseases. *Harefuah*. 2001 Dec;140(12):1 156–8, 1230.

38. Connor WE. n-3 Fatty acids from fish and fish oil: panacea or nostrum? *Am J Clin Nutr*. 2001 Oct;74(4):415–6.

39. Dewailly E, Blanchet C, Lemieux S et al. n-3 Fatty Acids and cardiovascular disease risk factors among the Inuit of Nunavik. *Am J Clin Nutr*. 2001 Oct;74(4):464–73.

40. Marchioli1 R. Dietary supplementation with n-3 polyunsaturated fatty acids and vitamin E after myocardial infarction:

results of the GISSI-Prevenzione trial. *Lancet.* 1999 Aug 7;354(9177):447–55.

41. von Schacky C, Angerer P, Kothny W, Theisen K, Mudra H. The effect of dietary omega-3 fatty acids on coronary atherosclerosis. A randomized, double-blind, placebo-controlled trial. *Ann Intern Med.* 1999 Apr 6;130(7):554–62.

42. Singh RB, Niaz MA, Sharma JP, Kumar R, Rastogi V, Moshiri M. Randomized, double-blind, placebo-controlled trial of fish oil and mustard oil in patients with suspected acute myocardial infarction: the Indian experiment of infarct survival-4. *Cardiovasc Drugs Ther.* 1997 Jul;1 1(3):485–91.

43. Das UN. Essential fatty acid metabolism in patients with essential hypertension, diabetes mellitus and coronary heart disease. *Prostaglandins Leukot Essent Fatty Acids.* 1995 Jun;52(6):387–91.

44. Garcia-Closas R, Serra-Majem L, Segura R. Fish consumption, omega-3 fatty acids and the Mediterranean diet. *Eur J Clin Nutr.* 1993 Sep;47 Suppl 1:S85–90.

45. Lukiw WJ, Cui JG, Marcheselli VL, et al. A role for docosahexaenoic acid-derived neuroprotectin D1 in neural cell survival and Alzheimer's disease. *J Clin Invest.* 2005 Oct;1 15(10):2774–83.

46. Bourre JM. Omega-3 fatty acids in psychiatry. *Med Sci* (Paris). 2005 Feb;21(2):216–21.

47. Bourre JM. Dietary omega-3 fatty acids and psychiatry: mood, behaviour, stress, depression, dementia and aging. *J Nutr Health Aging.* 2005 9(1):31–8.

48. Bourre JM. [The role of nutritional factors on the structure and function of the brain: an update on dietary requirements]. *Rev Neurol* (Paris). 2004 Sep;160(8–9):767–92.

49. Favreliere S, Perault MC, Huguet F, et al. DHA-enriched phospholipid diets modulate age-related alterations in rat hippocampus. *Neurobiol Aging.* 2003 Mar-Apr;24(2):233–43.

50. Martin DS, Lonergan PE, Boland B, et al. Apoptotic changes in the aged brain are triggered by interleukin-1 beta-induced activation of p38 and reversed by treatment with eicosapentaenoic acid. *J Biol Chem.* 2002 Sep 13;277(37):34239–46.

51. Youdim KA, Martin A, Joseph JA. Essential fatty acids and the brain: possible health implications. *Int J Dev Neurosci*. 2000 Jul-Aug; 1 8(4–5):383–99.

52. Conquer JA, Tierney MC, Zecevic J, Bettger WJ, Fisher RH. Fatty acid analysis of blood plasma of patients with Alzheimer's disease, other types of dementia, and cognitive impairment. *Lipids*. 2000 Dec;35(12):1305–12.

53. Morris MC, Evans DA, Bienias JL, et al. Consumption of fish and n-3 fatty acids and risk of incident Alzheimer's disease. *Arch Neurol*. 2003 Jul;60(7):940–6.

54. Kyle DJ, Schaefer E, Patton G, Beiser A. Low serum docosahexaenoic acid is a significant risk factor for Alzheimer's dementia. *Lipids*. 1999;34 Suppl:S245.

55. Hardman WE. n-3 fatty acids and cancer therapy. *J Nutr*. 2004 Dec;134(12 Suppl):3427S–430S.

56. Burns CP, Halabi S, Clamon GH, et al. Phase I clinical study of fish oil fatty acid capsules for patients with cancer cachexia: cancer and leukemia group B study 9473. *Clin Cancer Res*. 1999 Dec; 5(12):3942–7.

57. Tsuda H, Iwahori Y, Asamoto M, et al. Demonstration of organotropic effects of chemopreventive agents in multiorgan carcinogenesis models. *IARC Sci Publ*. 1996 (139):143–50.

58. Lai PB, Ross JA, Fearon KC, Anderson JD, Carter DC. Cell cycle arrest and induction of apoptosis in pancreatic cancer cells exposed to eicosapentaenoic acid in vitro. *Br J Cancer*. 1996 Nov;74(9):1375–83.

59. Gonzalez MJ. Fish oil, lipid peroxidation and mammary tumor growth. *J Am Coll Nutr*. 1995 Aug;14(4):325–35.

60. Zhu ZR, Agren J, Mannisto S, et al. Fatty acid composition of breast adipose tissue in breast cancer patients and patients with benign breast disease. *Nutr Cancer*. 1995;24(2):151–60.

61. O'Connor TP, Roebuck BD, Peterson F, Campbell TC. Effect of dietary intake of fish oil and fish protein on the development of L-azaserine-induced preneoplastic lesions in the rat pancreas. *J Natl Cancer Inst*. 1985 Nov;75(5):959–62.

FDA Threatens to Raid Cherry Orchards

A S AMERICANS STRUGGLE to eat a healthier diet, the FDA has taken draconian steps to suppress information about foods that reduce disease risk.

While various agencies of the federal government encourage us to eat more fruits and vegetables, the FDA has issued an edict that precludes cherry companies from posting scientific data on their websites. This censorship of published peer-reviewed studies denies consumers access to information that could be used to make wiser food choices.

Tobacco products kill 450,000 Americans each year.[1] Few people understand, however, that poor dietary habits are responsible for more deaths than tobacco. Considering the plethora of toxic foods advertised on television, it is easy to understand why so many consumers eat themselves to death. Just imagine if all you ate is what you saw advertised in the mass media.

The government stopped protecting the tobacco companies long ago, but the FDA continues to take actions that
steer Americans away from certain fruits and vegetables
that have proven disease-preventive effects.

FDA INTIMIDATES CHERRY GROWERS

There is not much profit in selling fresh fruits and vegetables. Growers of such foods cannot afford to advertise their
produce in a meaningful way. Fortunately, the advent of the
Internet has allowed cherry growers to enlighten the public
about scientific studies showing that nutrients contained in
cherries have significant health benefits.[2-15] Until recently,
consumers could learn of the health benefits of cherries just
by logging on to a cherry company's website. Some individuals might be impressed enough with this data to actually
buy cherries at the grocery store instead of trans fat-laden
snacks being advertised every second in the mass media.

On October 17, 2005, the FDA banned information
about cherries' health benefits from appearing on websites.[16,17] The FDA sent warning letters to 29 companies
that market cherry products. In these letters, the FDA
ordered the companies to stop publicizing scientific data
about cherries.[18] According to the FDA, when cherry companies disseminate this information, the cherries become
unapproved drugs subject to seizure. The FDA warns that
if those involved in cherry trafficking continue to inform
consumers about these scientific studies, criminal prose-
cutions will ensue.[17]

WHY AMERICANS DON'T EAT MORE FRUIT

The processed food industry has earned enormous profits
by loading cheap and dangerous foods with sugar, salt, pre-
servatives, trans fats, saturated fats, and other unhealthy

byproducts. Processed foods taste good to most people and are quite inexpensive compared to fresh produce. In order to convince the public to switch from toxic foods that damage the arterial wall, mutate DNA, and induce age-related disease, those who sell fresh fruits need to inform the public about the benefits scientists have discovered about plant foods.[19-37]

Fresh fruit can be expensive and it spoils relatively quickly. Many consumers have developed a taste addiction to processed foods, and find it challenging to switch to a healthier diet that costs more and is not as pleasing to the palate.

By censoring scientific information about cherries, the FDA is in effect shutting down an opportunity for more Americans to learn about the remarkable health benefits that have been discovered about this fruit.

DO CHERRIES PREVENT CANCER?

In a warning letter to Friske Orchards of Ellsworth, MI, the FDA recites the following information contained on this orchard's website:[38] "Tart cherries may reduce the risk of colon cancer because of the anthocyanins and cyanidin contained in the cherry."

The FDA goes on to say in its warning letter:

> These claims cause your product to be a drug as defined in section 201(g). . . . Because this product is not generally recognized as safe and effective when used as labeled, it is also defined as a new drug in section 201(p). . . . Under section 505 of the Act (21 USC 355), a new drug may not be legally marketed in the United States without an approved New Drug Application. . . .

Interestingly, the FDA is not denying the veracity of this information. Instead, it insists that a new drug application has to be approved before the public can be informed about the scientific data supporting cherries. The FDA also asserts, without any basis, that cherries "have not been recognized as safe and effective when used as labeled."[38] According to the FDA's interpretation of the law, cherry growers are engaged in criminal conduct by relaying findings that have been published in peer-reviewed scientific journals. Whether you or other Americans develop cancer does not appear to be a consideration of an agency whose written mission statement includes the following:

> The FDA is responsible for advancing the public health by helping to speed innovations that make medicines and foods more effective, safer, and more affordable; and helping the public get the accurate, science-based information they need to use medicines and foods to improve their health.[39]

As Life Extension® documented many years ago, the FDA does the opposite of what it pretends to do. Instead of "helping the public get the accurate, science-based information they need to use foods to improve their health," the FDA has gone to extreme lengths to deny American citizens the right to learn about scientific studies substantiating the health benefits discovered about cherries (and other fruits).

A MEDICAL ATROCITY!

In November 2004, Dr. David Graham, associate director for science at the FDA's Office of Drug Safety, testified before Congress that Vioxx® had caused 88,000 to 139,000 excess cases of heart attack and stroke.[40] Dr. Graham severely criticized his own employer (the FDA) for intentionally covering up information about the lethal side effects of Vioxx®.

The FDA is greatly concerned that cherry companies are disseminating scientific data showing that cherries are more effective than FDA-approved drugs in alleviating arthritis inflammation and pain.

The FDA is willing to throw cherry growers in jail for suggesting that their fruit may safely alleviate arthritis discomfort, yet the irrefutable facts are that the FDA intentionally concealed the dangers of Vioxx® for years, thereby causing the needless death of tens of thousands of Americans. Who are the real criminals here?

The FDA says it is responsible for "protecting the public health" by assuring the safety of drugs. It does not take much brainpower to see that the FDA's purported mission is nothing more than a hoax to protect the economic interests of the pharmaceutical giants.

It would appear that the FDA is concerned that if too many arthritis sufferers discover that eating cherries could alleviate inflammation and pain, the multibillion-dollar market for anti-inflammatory drugs would be detrimentally affected. Pharmaceutical industry profits have been spared for the moment by the flagrant acts perpetrated against cherry companies by the FDA.

CONGRESS RECOGNIZES PROBLEMS WITH FDA

As this nation faces a worsening healthcare crisis that threatens to bankrupt corporations, aging adults, and the government itself, members of Congress are becoming incensed that the FDA is suppressing proven methods to prevent and treat disease.

On November 10, 2005, a bill was introduced in the United States House of Representatives that would prohibit the FDA from denying consumers access to truthful health information. The name of this bill is the Health Freedom Protection Act (H.R. 4282).[41]

The original sponsors of this bill introduced it by exposing the FDA's inappropriate censorship of life-saving scientific information. Here is an excerpt from this historic speech:

> Because of the FDA's censorship of truthful health claims, millions of Americans may suffer with diseases and other healthcare problems they may have avoided by using dietary supplements. For example, the FDA prohibited consumers from learning how folic acid reduces the risk of neural tube defects for four years after the Centers for Disease Control and Prevention recommended every woman of childbearing age take folic acid supplements to reduce neural tube defects. This FDA action contributed to an estimated 10,000 cases of preventable neural tube defects!

> The FDA also continues to prohibit consumers from learning about the scientific evidence that glucosamine and chondroitin sulfate are effective in the treatment of osteoarthritis; that omega-3 fatty acids may reduce the risk of sudden death heart attack; and that calcium may reduce the risk of bone fractures.

> The Health Freedom Protection Act will force the FDA to at last comply with the commands of Congress, the First Amendment, and the American people by codifying the First Amendment standards adopted by the federal courts. Specifically, the Health Freedom Protection Act stops

the FDA from censoring truthful claims about the curative, mitigative, or preventative effects of dietary supplements, and adopts the federal court's suggested use of disclaimers as an alternative to censorship. The Health Freedom Protection Act also stops the FDA from prohibiting the distribution of scientific articles and publications regarding the role of nutrients in protecting against disease.[42]

CITIZENS REVOLT AGAINST BUREAUCRATIC CORRUPTION

When Life Extension® stated in 1989 that the law had to be changed to allow scientific information about foods and supplements to be freely disseminated, everyone told us that it was impossible to beat the entrenched FDA on Capitol Hill. As we went on national television and radio shows in the early 1990s to expose the incompetence and fraud perpetrated against the public by the FDA, a growing number of health-conscious individuals began to realize the magnitude of the problem.

In October 1994, by a nearly unanimous margin, Congress enacted the Dietary Supplement Health and Education Act (DSHEA), which allowed the public to learn about some of the health benefits attributed to certain nutrients.[43]

Despite significant losses in the federal courts regarding how DSHEA should be interpreted, the FDA is continuing to dedicate substantial resources to suppressing scientific information about how certain foods may prevent and treat disease. The FDA's arrogance is appalling in light of the record number of prescription drugs that have been withdrawn because too many users are dying from side effects. In the case of cherries, many of the scientific studies the FDA is concerned about relate to this fruit's anti-arthritic effect.[4-6,44,45]

The FDA's flagrant disregard for the First Amendment and DSHEA is one reason why the Health Freedom Protection Act was introduced. Members of Congress and the American public are fed up with the abuse of power perpetrated by an agency whose track record shows a reckless disregard for human life.

DRUG COMPANIES CONTROL FDA

The FDA has come under fire by the media and Congress for its failure to protect consumers against dangerous drugs. Life Extension® has long contended that large drug companies exert tremendous influence over the FDA. The result is that toxic drugs remain on the market while the sale of dietary supplements (and now even cherries) is impeded by FDA.

One reason doctors prescribe dangerous drugs is that pharmaceutical companies persuade the FDA to omit information concerning side effects from the drug's label. An egregious example of the incestuous control that drug companies exert over the FDA came to light with the Vioxx® scandal.

Based on evidence showing increased heart attack rates in Vioxx® users, the FDA suggested putting a cardiovascular warning on the label. Merck, the maker of Vioxx®, vehemently objected. On November 8, 2001, when talks with the FDA were not going to Merck's liking, the head of Merck's research department sent an email to his top scientists stating:

> Twice in my life I have had to say to the FDA, "That label is unacceptable, we will not under

any circumstances accept it." . . . I assure you I will NOT sign off on any label that has a cardiac warning for Vioxx®.[46]

Vioxx® was withdrawn from the market on September 30, 2004, after a clinical trial showed the risk of heart attack and stroke doubled for patients taking Vioxx® for more than 18 months.[47-49] The FDA knew about the cardiovascular risks of Vioxx® years before it was withdrawn, but succumbed to drug company pressure to omit this information from the drug's warning box. It did appear many months later on the label's "precautions box," which is normally too voluminous for anyone to read.

The statement by the Merck official that he would "not under any circumstances accept" a cardiovascular warning on Vioxx® provides a startling glimpse into how much control drug companies have over the FDA. Consumers are relegated to ingest toxic drugs while the FDA takes extraordinary measures to censor information showing the anti-arthritis efficacy of cherries.

UPDATE

As with many bills introduced that would give consumers access to truthful information about healthy foods and supplements, the Health Freedom Protection Act was not enacted into law by Congress, which is why FDA is able to censor truthful health claims about walnuts, green tea, and other foods that decrease disease risk.

References

1. Available at: http://www.cdc.gov/tobacco/factsheets/Tobacco_Related_Mortality_factsheet.htm. Accessed December 12, 2005.

2. Kang SY, Seeram NP, Nair MG, Bourquin LD. Tart cherry anthocyanins inhibit tumor development in Apc(Min) mice and reduce proliferation of human colon cancer cells. *Cancer Lett.* 2003 May 8;194(1):13–9.

3. Pratico D, Tillmann C, Zhang ZB, Li H, FitzGerald GA. Acceleration of atherogenesis by COX-1-dependent prostanoid formation in low density lipoprotein receptor knockout mice. *Proc Natl Acad Sci USA.* 2001 Mar 13;98(6):3358–63.

4. Tall JM, Seeram NP, Zhao C, et al. Tart cherry anthocyanins suppress inflammation-induced pain behavior in rat. *Behav Brain Res.* 2004 Aug 12;153(1):181–8.

5. Wang H, Nair MG, Strasburg GM, et al. Cyclooxygenase active bioflavonoids from Balaton tart cherry and their structure activity relationships. *Phytomedicine.* 2000 Mar;7(1):15–9.

6. Seeram NP, Momin RA, Nair MG, Bourquin LD. Cyclooxygenase inhibitory and antioxidant cyanidin glycosides in cherries and berries. *Phytomedicine.* 2001 Sep;8(5):362–9.

7. Wang H, Nair MG, Strasburg GM, et al. Antioxidant and anti-inflammatory activities of anthocyanins and their aglycon, cyanidin, from tart cherries. *J Nat Prod.* 1999 Feb;62(2):294–6.

8. Kolayli S, Kucuk M, Duran C, Candan F, Dincer B. Chemical and antioxidant properties of Laurocerasus officinalis Roem. (cherry laurel) fruit grown in the Black Sea region. *J Agric Food Chem.* 2003 Dec 3;51(25):7489–94.

9. Wakabayashi H, Fukushima H, Yamada T, et al. Inhibition of LPS-stimulated NO production in mouse macrophage-like cells by Barbados cherry, a fruit of Malpighia emarginata DC. *AntiCancer Res.* 2003 Jul;23(4):3237–41.

10. Nagamine I, Akiyama T, Kainuma M, et al. Effect of acerola cherry extract on cell proliferation and activation of ras signal pathway at the promotion stage of lung tumorigenesis in mice. *J Nutr Sci Vitaminol* (Tokyo). 2002 Feb;48(1):69–72.

11. Jacob RA, Spinozzi GM, Simon VA, et al. Consumption of cherries lowers plasma urate in healthy women. *J Nutr.* 2003 Jun;133(6):1826–9.

12. Rimm EB, Katan MB, Ascherio A, Stampfer MJ, Willett WC. Relation between intake of flavonoids and risk for coronary heart disease in male health professionals. *Ann Intern Med.* 1996 Sep 1;125(5):384–9.

13. Burkhardt S, Tan DX, Manchester LC, Hardeland R, Reiter RJ. Detection and quantification of the antioxidant melatonin in Montmorency and Balaton tart cherries (Prunus cerasus). *J Agric Food Chem.* 2001 Oct;49(10):4898–902.

14. Available at: http://pubs.acs.org/pressrelease/jafc/release3.html. Accessed December 15, 2005.

15. Available at: http://www.wholehealthmd.com/print/view/1,1560,SU_10015,00.html. Accessed December 15, 2005.

16. Available at: http://www.wjla.com/news/stories/1005/272655.html. Accessed December 15, 2005.

17. Available at: http://www.fda.gov/bbs/topics/news/2005/new01246.html. Accessed December 15, 2005.

18. Available at: http://www.cfsan.fda.gov/~dms/chrylist.html. Accessed December 15, 2005.

19. Available at: http://aspartametruth.com/ blaylock/interaction.html. Accessed December 15, 2005.

20. Available at: http://www.inmotionmagazine.com/ geff4.html. Accessed December 15, 2005.

21. Sasso FC, Carbonara O, Nasti R, et al. Glucose metabolism and coronary heart disease in patients with normal glucose tolerance. *JAMA.* 2004 Apr 21;291(15):1857–63.

22. Reiser S. Effect of dietary sugars on metabolic risk factors associated with heart disease. *Nutr Health.* 1985;3(4):203–16.

23. Pamplona R, Bellmunt MJ, Portero M, Prat J. Mechanisms of glycation in atherogenesis. *Med Hypotheses.* 1993 Mar;40 (3):174–81.

24. Reyes FG, Valim MF, Vercesi AE. Effect of organic synthetic food colours on mitochondrial respiration. *Food Addit Contam.* 1996 Jan;13(1):5–11.

25. Jagerstad M, Skog K. Genotoxicity of heat-processed foods. *Mutat Res*. 2005 Jul 1;574(1–2):156–72.

26. Sasaki YF, Kawaguchi S, Kamaya A, et al. The comet assay with 8 mouse organs: results with 39 currently used food additives. *Mutat Res*. 2002 Aug 26;519(1–2): 103–19.

27. Tsuda S, Murakami M, Matsusaka N, et al. DNA damage induced by red food dyes orally administered to pregnant and male mice. *Toxicol Sci*. 2001 May;61(1):92–9.

28. Ashida H, Hashimoto T, Tsuji S, Kanazawa K, Danno G. Synergistic effects of food colors on the toxicity of 3-amino-1,4¬dimethyl-5H-pyrido[4,3-b]indole (Trp-P-1) in primary cultured rat hepatocytes. *J Nutr Sci Vitaminol* (Tokyo). 2000 Jun;46(3):130–6.

29. Tjaderhane L, Larmas M. A high sucrose diet decreases the mechanical strength of bones in growing rats. *J Nutr*. 1998 Oct;128(10):1807–10.

30. Veromann S, Sunter A, Tasa G, et al. Dietary sugar and salt represent real risk factors for cataract development. *Ophthalmologica*. 2003 Jul;217(4):302–7.

31. Michaud DS, Liu S, Giovannucci E, et al. Dietary sugar, glycemic load, and pancreatic cancer risk in a prospective study. *J Natl Cancer Inst*. 2002 Sep 4;94(17):1293–300.

32. Molteni R, Barnard RJ, Ying Z, Roberts CK, Gomez-Pinilla F. A high-fat, refined sugar diet reduces hippocampal brain-derived neurotrophic factor, neuronal plasticity, and learning. *Neuroscience*. 2002;112(4):803–14.

33. Blacklock NJ. Sucrose and idiopathic renal stone. *Nutr Health*. 1987;5(1–2):9–17.

34. Moerman CJ, Bueno de Mesquita HB, Runia S. Dietary sugar intake in the aetiology of biliary tract cancer. *Int J Epidemiol*. 1993 Apr;22(2):207–14.

35. Kruis W, Forstmaier G, Scheurlen C, Stellaard F. Effect of diets low and high in refined sugars on gut transit, bile acid metabolism, and bacterial fermentation. *Gut*. 1991 Apr;32(4):367–71.

36. Yudkin J, Eisa O. Dietary sucrose and oestradiol concentration in young men. *Ann Nutr Metab*. 1988;32(2):53–5.

37. De Stefani E, Deneo-Pellegrini H, Mendilaharsu M, Ronco A, Carzoglio JC. Dietary sugar and lung cancer: a case-control study in Uruguay. *Nutr Cancer*. 1998;31(2):132–7.
38. Available at: http://www.fda.gov/foi/warning_letters/g5531d.htm. Accessed December 15, 2005.
39. Available at: http://www.fda.gov/opacom/morechoices/mission.html. Accessed December 15, 2005.
40. Available at: http://www.finance.senate.gov/ sitepages/ hearing111804.htm. Accessed December 15, 2005.
41. Available at: http://thomas.loc.gov/. Accessed December 15, 2005.
42. Available at: http://www.house.gov/ paul/congrec/congrec2005/cr111005.htm. Accessed December 15, 2005.
43. Available at: http://www.fda.gov/opacom/laws/dshea.html. Accessed December 15, 2005.
44. Available at: http://www.arthritis.org/resources/arthritistoday/2002_archives/2002_09_10_OnCall.asp. Accessed December 15, 2005.
45. Blando F, Gerardi C, Nicoletti I. Sour cherry (Prunus cerasus L) anthocyanins as ingredients for functional foods. *J Biomed Biotechnol*. 2004;2004(5):253–8.
46. Martinez B. Novartis fights eczema drug's cancer warning. *Wall Street Journal*. April 8, 2005.
47. Bresalier RS, Sandler RS, Quan H, et al. Cardiovascular events associated with rofecoxib in a colorectal adenoma chemoprevention trial. *N Engl J Med*. 2005 Mar 17;352(11):1092–102.
48. Topol EJ. Failing the public healthrofecoxib, Merck, and the FDA. *N Engl J Med*. 2004 Oct 21;351(17):1707–9.
49. Martinez B. Merck documents shed light on Vioxx® legal battles. *Wall Street Journal*. February 7, 2005

2005

Inside the FDA's Brain

THE FDA HAS RELEASED a detailed report that states, "it is highly unlikely that green tea reduces the risk of prostate cancer."[1]

The FDA made it clear that it evaluates lots of evidence when deciding whether to allow a health claim. Most of this evidence, however, is eliminated from further review because it does not meet the agency's standards.

While there are numerous published studies on green tea and prostate cancer, the FDA determined that only two met its standards. The first study cited by the agency showed that drinking three cups of green tea a day reduced prostate cancer risk by 73%.[2] The second study did not provide statistically significant data, but showed that drinking two to 10 cups of green tea daily reduced prostate cancer risk by 33%.[3] According to the FDA, "both studies received high methodological quality ratings."

Based on these two human studies, the FDA will allow the following health claim for green tea beverages:

One weak and limited study does not show that drinking green tea reduces the risk of prostate cancer, but another weak and limited study suggests that drinking green tea may reduce this risk. Based on these studies, FDA concludes that it is highly unlikely that green tea reduces the risk of prostate cancer.[1]

WHY FDA CALLS THESE "WEAK" STUDIES

The FDA's gold standard is tightly controlled studies that consist of an active component and a placebo arm. The two green tea studies chosen by the FDA evaluated the effects of historical consumption of green tea beverages on prostate cancer risk.

The studies showed that the greater the consumption of green tea, the lower the prostate cancer risk. This does not, however, impress the FDA as much as a carefully designed study where half of the men would drink three to 10 cups of green tea a day while the other half drank a placebo beverage.

While the FDA admits that the study showing a 73% reduction in prostate cancer risk is significant, the agency believes the study that showed a non-statistically significant 33% risk reduction cancelled out the better study. According to the FDA, "replication of scientific findings is important in order to substantiate results."[4,5]

THE OMITTED STUDY

While the FDA claims to have extensively reviewed the scientific literature to find the truth about green tea and prostate cancer, one important study was overlooked.

In a tightly controlled clinical setting, men with premalignant prostate disease were given either 600 mg a day of green tea extract or a placebo. Compared to those who received the placebo, men with this pre-malignant condition who received the green tea extract were 90% less likely to develop prostate cancer.[6]

While the FDA may argue that green tea supplements differ from green tea beverages, the fact is that this placebo-controlled study existed, but was omitted from the FDA's report. The FDA's report concluded:

> Based on FDA's review of the strength of the total body of publicly available scientific evidence for a claim about green tea and reduced risk of prostate cancer, FDA ranks this evidence as the lowest level for a qualified health claim. For the reasons given above, FDA concludes that it is highly unlikely that green tea reduces the risk of prostate cancer.[4]

THE FDA PRESS RELEASE

The FDA issued a press release to alert the world that green tea has little or no value in preventing cancer. The news media picked up on the FDA's negative findings about green tea and echoed the agency's claims that green tea does not prevent cancer.

Newspapers and television stations reported that consumers were wasting their money by drinking green tea. None of these media sources bothered to check the National Library of Medicine's database to find over 600 studies relating to green tea and cancer. Even a cursory review of these studies reveals a very different story than what was contained in the FDA's press release.

The National Library of Medicine is part of the US Department of Health and Human Services, the same parent agency as the FDA!

CONSUMERS NEED TO KNOW THE FACTS

The United States faces a worsening healthcare crisis as aging baby boomers financially exhaust the nation's medical systems.

The FDA is empowered to regulate almost every aspect of our healthcare, yet this federal agency continues to behave in a manner that promotes illness. An unbiased review of the published scientific literature reveals health properties attributed to green tea, but the FDA has restricted what Americans are allowed to read on the labels of green tea beverages.

If the data about green tea and prostate cancer risk turn out to be only partially accurate, the lives of millions of men could be saved and billions of dollars shaved off future healthcare expenditures. Yet the law still allows the FDA to censor truthful information about foods and dietary supplements.

WE CAN CHANGE THE LAW

On May 12, 2005, a bill was introduced in the US House of Representatives that would give consumers access to truthful, non-misleading health information. This bill— the Consumers' Access to Health Information Act (H.R. 2352)[7]—seeks to amend the Food, Drug and Cosmetic Act to ensure that:

- Accurate health claims are not suppressed;
- Consumers are given truthful and complete information about the curative, mitigation, treatment, and prevention effects of foods and dietary supplements on disease or health-related conditions;
- The FDA honors the intent of the Congress not to censor accurate health claims.

This is one of the most critical pieces of legislation to ever come before Congress. Passage of the Consumers' Access to Health Information Act would enable the American public to learn how to prevent many of the degenerative diseases of aging. This bill could help avert the healthcare crisis that is threatening to bankrupt Medicare, corporations, and aging adults.

UPDATE

An apathetic Congress again failed to pass this bill (Consumer's Access to Health Information Act) that would have enabled Americans to learn about the disease prevention potential of healthy dietary practices.

References

1. FDA issues information for consumers about claims for green tea and certain cancers [press release]. Washington, DC: US Food and Drug Administration; June 30, 2005.

2. Jian L, Xie LP, Lee AH, Binns CW. Protective effect of green tea against prostate cancer: a case-control study in southeast China. *Int J Cancer*. 2004 Jan 1;108(1):130–5.

3. Sonoda T, Nagata Y, Mori M et al. A case-control study of diet and prostate cancer in Japan: possible protective effect of traditional Japanese diet. *Cancer Sci*. 2004 Mar;95(3):238–42.

4. Available at: http://www.cfsan.fda.gov/~dms/qhc-gtea.html. Accessed August 19, 2005.

5. Wilson EB Jr. Replication of scientific findings is important for evaluating the strength of scientific evidence. In: *An Introduction to Scientific Research*. Mineola, NY: Dover Publications;1990:46–48.

6. Available at: http://www.aacr.org/Default.aspx?p=1066&d=432. Accessed August 19, 2005.

7. Available at: http://thomas.loc.gov/cgi-bin/query/z?c109:H.R.2352.IH. Accessed August 19, 2005.

FDA Fails to Protect Domestic Drug Supply

I F YOU TAKE THE INFORMATION on the FDA's website at face value, you would be convinced that the FDA has guaranteed the safety of our drug supply—as long as you do not import any prescription drugs from outside the United States.

According to the FDA's website, medications not approved for sale in the US may not have been manufactured under this nation's rigid quality assurance procedures that ensure a safe, effective product. These imported drugs may not have been evaluated for safety and effectiveness in the US, and thus might be addictive or even contain dangerous substances. Moreover, according to the FDA's website, some imported medications—even those bearing the name of a US-approved product—may be counterfeit versions that are unsafe or even completely ineffective. The FDA suggests that you need not worry about these dangers if you buy drugs from domestic pharmacies.[1]

Joe McCallion, a consumer safety officer in the FDA's Office of Regulatory Affairs, sums it up this way: "If you buy drugs that come from outside the US, the FDA doesn't know what you're getting, which means safety can't be assured."[1]

On the other hand, the FDA website notes that drugs sold in the US must be made in accordance with good manufacturing practices, and all products must have proper labeling that conforms to FDA requirements. As part of the FDA's "high" standards, drugs can be manufactured only at plants registered with the agency, and manufacturers are subject to ongoing FDA inspections. Along with these legal requirements, US pharmacists and wholesalers must be licensed or authorized in the states where they operate.[1] These safeguards in the process of getting drugs onto US pharmacy shelves ensure that the products you buy are safe and effective.

It is a great argument, designed to assure us that the FDA has things well under control. If only it were true.

THE REAL STORY

In fact, the drugs you buy pass through a network of wholesalers operating under lax state supervision and virtually no FDA supervision. You probably assume the drug manufacturers ship their products directly to pharmacies, maintaining strict control all along the way. Not so. Big pharmaceutical companies use middlemen that buy, sell, sort, repackage, and distribute 98% of the nation's medicine. These middlemen, numbering about 6,500 in all, range from publicly traded giants with pristine warehouses to small, obscure, backroom operators. While the three largest companies control 90% of this market, below them are some 15 regional wholesalers, and below them are scores of smaller secondary wholesalers.

All of these middlemen, regardless of size, aim to buy medicine as cheaply as possible and resell it for a profit, a system of arbitrage made possible by widely varying drug prices. Drug companies offer an array of targeted discounts that result in their selling the exact same drug for any number of prices.

These varying prices often spark frenetic trading among the wholesalers. The "Big Three" distributors have trading divisions that scout the secondary wholesale market for discounted medicine, and they have been known to boast how much they saved by purchasing heavily discounted medicine from obscure wholesalers. The secondary wholesalers contend that this aggressive trading helps reduce drug prices for mom-and-pop pharmacies and local hospitals that lack the buying power of the big chains.

However, the bargains also drive a parallel and illegal process called diversion, in which some middlemen resort to fraud or misrepresentation to obtain discounted medicine. Corrupt wholesalers often solicit "closed-door" pharmacies (those that supposedly buy only for themselves) and others that qualify for discounts to buy more medicine than they need and sell the rest out the back door for kickbacks. In 2000, the National Association of Boards of Pharmacy estimated that up to four-fifths of the closed-door pharmacies that received discounted medicine illegally resold at least a portion of it to outside buyers.

STOLEN DRUGS

In her book, *Dangerous Doses: How Counterfeiters Are Contaminating America's Drug Supply*, investigative medical reporter Katherine Eban details the results of a two-year exploration of America's secret ring of drug counterfeiters, following the trail of medicine as it winds its way from a seemingly minor break-in to a sprawling national network of drug polluters. She follows the progress of a team of Florida criminal investigators as they uncover sickening examples of stolen medicine that is resold as the genuine article without any of the safeguards we assume exist for prescription drugs.[2]

While the FDA has an Office of Criminal Investigations, the agency does not aggressively pursue these matters. The wholesalers profiled in *Dangerous Doses* use this confusion to their advantage. They have state licenses, lawyers, accountants, and all the trappings of legitimacy. Their goal is to buy low, sell high, and make money. But they have little incentive to maintain drugs in pristine condition.[2]

Three years ago in Florida, it was laughably easy to become a pharmaceutical wholesaler. All you needed was a refrigerator, an air conditioner, an alarm to secure your products, $200 for a security bond, and $700 for a license. No experience or particular knowledge was required. You had to certify that you had no criminal record, but the state's pharmaceutical bureau did not actually check for a criminal background. Through this loophole slipped all sorts of unsavory characters: former cocaine dealers looking for good money with less chance of jail time, real estate hucksters, and others. Once established, a pharmaceutical wholesaler had little reason to worry about FDA inspections. State authorities alone regulated your business. And each inspector had some 300 companies to look after.[2]

With this regulatory framework, Florida's pharmaceutical wholesale companies proliferated like rabbits, far beyond any need for them. By 2002, Florida had licensed 1,399 wholesalers, one for every three pharmacies in the state. The vast majority of these companies were based out of state, though some actually were Florida operations. The wholesalers set up "corporate headquarters" by rerouting their calls and faxes to make it appear that they had offices everywhere.[2]

Not surprisingly, criminal elements were drawn to this regulatory vacuum like moths to a flame. The state investigation began when a two-bit burglar stole cancer medicine from an unlocked refrigerator at Jackson Memorial Hospital in Miami. Caught in the act, he cooperated with police in return for leniency, agreeing to carry a hidden microphone while he sold his stolen goods. The woman who bought the drug, a licensed wholesaler, threw it in the hot trunk of her car while she did errands, destroying the potency of this delicate medicine without any obvious indication of damage. According to the investigators, this adulteration happens frequently, with the end-user of the drug being the hapless victim. Arrested later that day, she also agreed to cooperate, and in time the state investigators worked their way to the kingpins of the trade, who were making millions from this illicit activity.[2]

RECYCLED DRUGS

One of these men was Michael Carlow, who pocketed $2.5 million in a single eight-month period. Duffel bags delivered to his house were filled with pill bottles, medicine vials, and bags of blood derivatives, all culled from different sources and some still bearing the labels of the patients to whom they had been dispensed.[2]

His conspirators maintained the flow of discounted inventory by buying anti-cancer and anti-AIDS drugs from patients treated at health clinics in Miami's slums. Some of those infected with HIV/AIDS were crack addicts who preferred getting high to getting well. Carlow's associates waited for them outside the clinics and swayed them to sell their Medicaid-supplied medicine (including growth hormone that retails for more than $1,000) for a few $20 bills.[2]

Carlow sold the medicine through his licensed wholesale businesses, using a variety of aliases to make them appear to be independently owned. The buyers of his goods would sometimes meet Carlow or an assistant at a gas station to exchange medicine for checks or cash. At Carlow's office, the state investigators found nail polish remover, lighter fluid, and paint remover cluttering the worktables and desks. The employees apparently used these products to remove patient dispensing labels and any other evidence of a product's origin. However, Carlow did not stop at selling to small, obscure companies. He developed a lucrative relationship with one of the Big Three distributors. In 2000, Carlow sold almost $2 million in contaminated or even counterfeit products to National Specialty Services, a Big Three division that at the time was the nation's largest supplier of blood products, cancer drugs, and other specialty pharmaceuticals to hospitals.[2]

STOLEN BLOOD

Carlow was not the only kingpin to be trapped in the state investigators' dragnet. In January 2002, thieves stole 344 vials of specialty blood products from a refrigerator in the warehouse of BioMed Plus, one of the nation's largest wholesale distributors of these drugs. These products, worth $335,000 wholesale, were destined for patients with compromised immune systems, hemophilia, and other rare disorders. Incredibly, the owner of BioMed Plus received a call a few days later from a wholesaler who offered to let him buy back a list of products identical to his list of stolen goods for a discounted price of $229,241. This medicine is rare and is almost never traded freely, so BioMed's owner knew the goods were his. He cooperated with investigators to retrieve the stolen drugs, but had to destroy the medicine because he could not guarantee that it had been properly stored during the heist.[2]

COUNTERFEIT DRUGS

The state investigators also discovered a filthy Miami warehouse filled with $15 million worth of counterfeit, diverted, and illegally re-imported medicine, as well as pill-making machines and 2 million tablets of counterfeit Lipitor®.

By the end of 2004, the state investigators had arrested 55 suspects—more than 30 of them on racketeering charges—and seized $33 million in bad medicine and almost $3 million in cash. Sixteen suspects agreed to cooperate, most pleading guilty to an array of charges. As a result of these state and local investigations, the Florida Legislature tightened its regulation of wholesalers, reducing their numbers by 50% (still one for every six pharmacies). Statewide Medicaid costs plunged for certain categories of drugs that had been overprescribed, billed to Medicaid, diverted to clinics, and prescribed again.[2]

Throughout the entire investigation, the FDA did nothing to help track down and bring these criminals to justice.

FDA FAILS TO PROTECT CONSUMERS

This story provides yet another example of how the FDA places the profits of drug companies and wholesalers above the health of the American consumer. The FDA has the authority to go after the counterfeiters and prosecute them aggressively. However, doing so would expose the current lack of safety to the glare of publicity, showing that the agency is not doing its job despite its power to do so. Far better to cast negative aspersions on the safety of imported drugs and allege that the supposed dangers are so great that we must construct a protective wall around our borders, within which pharmaceutical companies can charge a king's ransom for drugs available at a fraction of the price overseas.

When the author of *Dangerous Doses* called the public relations director of a major drug company to inform him that numerous lots of his company's lifesaving drug had been relabeled to appear 20 times their actual strength and that a licensed distributor was suspected of trafficking in counterfeit versions of that same medicine, his response was, "I'd hate to have you short the stock [try to profit from a decline in the share price] because of these local and contained incidents."[2] This outrageous response professes not anger at the possible contamination and threat to public health, but concern about a possible financial loss if word of the counterfeiting problem were to get out. Obviously, this executive's fear about the value of his stock options trumped any concern that people could suffer and perhaps die because of incidents that are by no means "local and contained."

It is bad enough that Americans have to pay an arm and a leg in the US for drugs that can be purchased for less money in Canada and Europe. Now, due to the investigative reporting in *Dangerous Doses* and the diligent efforts of Florida investigators, we are finding that drugs we purchase in the US may actually be more dangerous than those the FDA says we should not obtain from abroad.

The FDA pretends to protect consumers against contaminated drugs, but the sordid facts do not support this self-serving assertion. FDA complicity has enabled criminals to get potentially dangerous drugs into our local pharmacies.

References

1. Available at: http://www.fda.gov/fdac/features/2002/502_import.html. Accessed May 18, 2005.

2. Eban K. *Dangerous Doses: How Counterfeiters Are Contaminating America's Drug Supply*. Orlando, FL: Harcourt, Inc; 2005.

2004

FDA Permits New Fish Oil Health Claim

I**T WAS LONG AGO ESTABLISHED** that consumption of cold-water fish reduces the risk of heart attack.[1] In fact, just two to three servings of fish a week may protect against many diseases, including arthritis, stroke, certain cancers, and a host of inflammation-related disorders.[2-9]

When scientists sought to discover which components of fish are responsible for preventing heart attacks, they found that the oil plays a critical role. Coldwater fish oil is high in omega-3 fatty acids that function in multiple ways to reduce cardiovascular disease risk.[10]

Based on the published scientific evidence about fish oil, a lawsuit was filed against the FDA in 1994 by Durk Pearson and Sandy Shaw, seeking to force the agency to allow the following health claim on fish oil supplement labels: "Consumption of omega-3 fatty acids may reduce the risk of coronary heart disease." The FDA rejected this one-sentence claim and a multiyear litigation battle ensued.

In their lawsuit, Durk and Sandy pointed out that consumers would benefit by learning of the value of fish oil in protecting against heart disease. They also argued that the FDA lacked the constitutional authority to ban this truthful health claim.

The FDA contended that this health claim was not adequately backed by scientific studies and that the agency had the legal authority to ban these kinds of health claims.

Seven years of extensive litigation ensued as the FDA asserted that it had the sole authority to dictate what Americans could read on the label of fish oil supplements. After an onslaught of irrefutable scientific evidence was presented, including articles published in the most prestigious scientific journals in the world, the FDA capitulated and said it would permit the following claim:

> Consumption of omega-3 fatty acids may reduce the risk of coronary heart disease. FDA evaluated the data and determined that although there is scientific evidence supporting the claim, the evidence is not conclusive.

LIFE EXTENSION® CHALLENGES FDA ON FISH OIL HEALTH CLAIM

The FDA's compromise health claim that the evidence was "not conclusive" did not satisfy the Life Extension Foundation®. The scientific literature provided overwhelming validation that consuming coldwater fish or fish oils dramatically lowers heart attack risk.

To substantiate this position, a massive document enumerating the scientific studies backing the benefits of omega-3 fatty acids was filed, along with legal arguments supporting the constitutional right to disseminate this truthful information.

The Life Extension Foundation® Buyers Club, Inc., and Wellness Lifestyles, Inc., filed a health claim petition against the FDA on June 23, 2003. The petition urged the FDA to reconsider its permitted health claim for omega-3 fatty acids and coronary heart disease risk, and to allow the following revised claim: "Consumption of omega-3 fatty acids may reduce the risk of coronary heart disease."

Also included in the petition was a calculation of how many American lives were needlessly being lost because of the FDA's restriction of this simple health claim. Epidemiological data were presented showing that if all Americans regularly took fish oil supplements or ate about two cold-water fish meals a week, it would prevent about 150,000 deaths a year. Life Extension® further argued that during the seven years it took to litigate this case against the FDA, Americans suffered over 1 million preventable sudden-death heart attacks.

THE POLITICAL BATTLE OVER WHAT AMERICANS EAT

Junk food is big business in the United States. Processed food companies have historically used their political clout to persuade the federal government to defend the safety of dangerous food products. The cost of treating diseases caused by poor diet has become so staggering, however, that the government is recommending that Americans eat healthier.

For nearly two decades, the FDA protected the economic interests of companies selling high-fat and high-cholesterol foods by making it illegal to promote a healthy diet as a way of preventing heart disease. Sudden-death heart attacks were three times higher in the 1950s than in the 1990s. The FDA's censorship of healthy dietary information caused tens of millions of Americans to unnecessarily succumb to cardiovascular and other diseases.

FDA CAPITULATES TO SCIENTIFIC REALITY

On September 8, 2004, the FDA announced that it would allow an expanded health claim on products containing the omega-3 fatty acids eicosapentaenoic acid (EPA) and docosahexaenoic acid (DHA).

According to Acting FDA Commissioner Dr. Lester M. Crawford, "Coronary heart disease is a significant health problem that causes 500,000 deaths annually in the United States. This new qualified health claim for omega-3 fatty acids should help consumers as they work to improve their health by identifying foods that contain these important compounds (EPA and DHA)."

The FDA now permits the following statement to be printed on the label of fish oil supplements: "Supportive but not conclusive research shows that consumption of EPA and DHA omega-3 fatty acids may reduce the risk of coronary heart disease."

The FDA went on to recommend that consumers not exceed more than 3 grams per day of EPA and DHA omega-3 fatty acids, with no more than 2 grams per day derived from a dietary supplement. Life Extension® argues that many scientific studies show that higher amounts of EPA and DHA are often needed to obtain optimal benefits, such as reduction of triglycerides and prevention of restenosis (re-occlusion of a blocked artery).[11]

This battle over what can be stated about fish oil began back in 1994. While the FDA's announcement of a broader health claim represents a significant legal victory, Life Extension® is still not satisfied with the FDA's latest health claim on fish oil supplements. We reiterate our position that evidence from peer-reviewed scientific publications supporting the benefit of EPA and DHA supplements in reducing heart attack risk is conclusive and not merely "supportive" as the FDA contends.

Attorney Jonathan Emord put hundreds of hours of productive work into this case over the past ten years. Jonathan filed the initial lawsuit against the FDA on behalf of Durk Pearson and Sandy Shaw that resulted in a precedent-setting legal victory against FDA censorship. Jonathan then prepared the petition on behalf of Life Extension® and Wellness Lifestyles that resulted in the FDA allowing this new expanded health claim to be made about the protective effect of fish oils against cardiovascular disease.

UPDATE

Even though FDA claimed that Americans should not consume more than 2,000 mg a day of EPA/DHA from supplements when fish oil was approved as a prescription drug, far higher doses were allowed by FDA.

References

1. FTC Press Release, November 29, 2000. "FTC Reaches Record Price-fixing Settlement to Settle Charges of Price-fixing in Generic Drug Market."
2. Price quoted by Hollywood Discount Pharmacy in Hollywood, Florida on Jan 15, 2002.
3. Associated Press, October 4, 2001. "Drugmaker to pay $875 million fine."
4. Robert Pear (*New York Times* News Service). "Health spending jumps 6.9%—Main factors: hospitals and drug costs, managed care resistance, *The Herald*, Tuesday, January 8, 2002.
5. Faloon William, "Dying from Deficiency," *Life Extension Magazine*®, October 2001.
6. *National Vital Statistics Reports*, Vol. 48, No.11.
7. *Wall Street Journal*, December 24, 2001, pp-A3, "Schering Fines Could Total $500 Million."
8. http://www.cnn.com/HEALTH/9804/14/drug.reaction/Chicago CNN. "Study: Drug reactions kill an estimated 100,000 a year," April 14, 1998.

9. David Willman, "The Rise and Fall of the Killer Drug Rezulin," *Life Extension Magazine®*, September 2000.

10. http://news.ft.com/ft/gx.cgi/ftc?pagename= View&c=Article&cid=FT3HZ3AFMWC &live=true&tagid=IXL HT5GTICC&subheading=heal By David Firn in London, "More deaths linked to Bayer's Lipobay," January 18, 2002. 19:44. Last Updated: January 18 2002 19:48

11. Calder PC. n-3 fatty acids and cardiovascular disease: evidence explained and mechanisms explored. *Clin Sci* (Lond). 2004 Jul; 107(1): 1–11.

MAY 2004

FDA Approves Deadly Drugs, Delays Lifesaving Therapies

W HAT IF A DIETARY SUPPLEMENT was shown to kill 100 Americans and cause 56,000 emergency room visits each year?[1] Without a doubt, the supplement would be banned immediately and those who knowingly marketed such a lethal product would be subject to severe criminal penalties.

On January 22, 2004, the FDA confirmed that acetaminophen is extremely dangerous.[2] Acetaminophen is sold under the brand name Tylenol® and is contained in 600 other drug products. The toxicity of acetaminophen was clear more than 12 years ago, and *Life Extension®* harshly criticized the FDA for not mandating that the label of acetaminophen products warn those with liver or kidney problems to avoid the drug.

In 2002, an FDA scientific advisory committee urged that warnings be put on the labels of acetaminophen drugs.[3,4] Despite overwhelming documentation confirming acetaminophen's toxicity,[5-28] the FDA said no to its own scientific advisors. Instead, the agency has budgeted a mere $20,000[29,30] to develop material that it hopes will be run in major magazines and distributed by pharmacy chains for free! This is the bureaucratic equivalent of doing nothing.

The agency spends tens of millions of dollars a year attacking companies selling natural health products that have harmed no one. Yet the FDA is making virtually no effort to prevent the 100 deaths and 56,000 emergency room visits that the agency itself admits are caused by acetaminophen drugs every year![31]

ACETAMINOPHEN RISKS UNDERSTATED

Back in 1992, research showed that many more people are dying because of acetaminophen than the number indicated by the official statistics. While the FDA was preoccupied with acetaminophen-induced liver failure, it overlooked studies showing that regular users of acetaminophen may be doubling their risk of kidney cancer.[11,13,32]

What does that translate to in actual numbers of victims? Each year, almost 12,000 Americans die of kidney cancer.[33] The incidence of kidney cancer in the US has risen 126% since the 1950s,[34] a jump that may be tied to the growing use of drugs containing phenacetin or acetaminophen.

Phenacetin is a painkiller that was banned because it causes severe kidney toxicity.[35-40] Acetaminophen is the major metabolite of phenacetin, which means that some of the destructive properties exhibited by phenacetin could have been caused by its breakdown to acetaminophen in the body. So while phenacetin was withdrawn because too many people's kidneys were shutting down, the FDA had no problem letting the major metabolite of phenacetin (acetaminophen) be freely marketed without any consumer warning whatsoever.

If acetaminophen is responsible for even a small percentage of the overall kidney cancer cases, this drug may have already killed tens of thousands of Americans—and the FDA has done nothing to stop this carnage!

Because acetaminophen generates damaging free radicals throughout the body, it may very well increase the risk of many age-related diseases. In fact, scientists can consistently induce cataracts in the eyes of laboratory animals by giving them acetaminophen. They consider acetaminophen a "cataratogenic agent." Interestingly, if antioxidants are provided to the animals, the cataract-inducing effects of acetaminophen are often completely neutralized.[41-46]

The antioxidant N-acetylcysteine helps neutralize destructive free radicals. When a person acutely overdoses on acetaminophen, the standard medical therapy is to administer N-acetylcysteine over a period of weeks. Unfortunately, the FDA bans the combination of an over-the-counter drug (acetaminophen) with a dietary supplement (N-acetylcysteine), so it is "illegal" to make a safe acetaminophen drug.

Despite the overwhelming evidence that acetaminophen use should be strictly limited, the FDA capitulates to pharmaceutical companies that earn billions of dollars a year selling this lethal class of analgesic drug.

By failing to mandate a warning on the label of acetaminophen products, the FDA once again demonstrates its propensity for protecting the pharmaceutical industry's economic interests at the expense of the American public's health.

FDA DENIES ALZHEIMER'S DRUG FOR 14 YEARS

At any given time, 4 million Americans suffer the devastating consequences of Alzheimer's disease.[47] Alzheimer's has no cure, and all victims suffer a progressive neurodegenerative process that results in total disability and death.

In 1990, a drug used in Germany was found to slow the progression of the disease.[48] The drug's generic name is memantine, and Life Extension® has long recommended it to family members of Alzheimer's victims.[49]

Memantine does not offer miraculous benefits. The studies show that some patients experience improvements in memory and cognitive skills.[50] For the vast majority, however, memantine merely slows the pace of deterioration, enabling patients to perform certain functions a little longer than would otherwise be possible.[51,52] For example, the drug enabled some patients to go to the bathroom independently for an additional six months, a benefit caregivers called very important.[53]

The July 2001 issue of *Life Extension*® featured an in-depth report on the clinical value of memantine in treating a wide range of disorders, including Parkinson's disease, glaucoma, and diabetic neuropathy.[54] It was highly critical of the FDA's attempts to deny Alzheimer's patients residing in the US access to this safe and partially effective medication.

Starting this year, Americans can purchase memantine sold under the brand name Namenda® at American pharmacies. One reason memantine is available now is the intense pressure put on the FDA by family members of Alzheimer's victims who had to order the drug from Europe and risk FDA seizure.

Americans had to wait 14 years to gain legal access to a drug proven to work in Europe. In 1991, the FDA was sued for denying access to the drug tacrine for Alzheimer's patients. Tacrine's mechanism of action inhibits the ace-tylcholinesterase enzyme, thus making more of the neu-rotransmitter acetylcholine available to brain cells. Six months after the lawsuit was dropped, the FDA approved tacrine.[55] And few years later still, the FDA approved a safer drug called Aricept® that shares some of tacrine's same mechanisms of action but is less toxic.[56]

Memantine works by a different mechanism than tacrine or Aricept®. Memantine blocks a reaction known as "excitotoxicity," a pathological process in which too much glutamate is released in the brain, severely damag-ing the neurons. Those seeking to protect their healthy neurons against the damaging effects of excitotoxicity use dietary supplements such as methylcobalamin and vinpocetine. That it took litigation, harsh media criti-cism, and a citizens' uprising to motivate the FDA to approve these Alzheimer's drugs is a testament to the agency's inability to differentiate between safe, effective medications that should be approved and lethal drugs that should be removed .[57]

WHO WILL PROTECT US FROM THE FDA?

The FDA pretends to protect Americans from dangerous and ineffective products, yet even a cursory review of the agency's track record reveals the opposite to be true. Dan-gerous and ineffective drugs are approved, while novel lifesaving therapies and natural approaches to disease prevention are brutally suppressed.[58-69]

The FDA's failure to mandate a warning on the label of acetaminophen products is just one example of its failure to protect consumers against lethal drug side effects. The agency's inexcusable delay in approving drugs to allevi-ate the miseries of Alzheimer's disease reveals its lack of compassion for human beings who have lost the cognitive ability to take care of themselves.

Since 1980, the Life Extension Foundation® has recommended drugs that the FDA has not yet approved.[70-73] In many cases, what we recommended was eventually approved, which means that our scientific analysis—as opposed to the FDA's politically motivated decision-making process—was medically correct.

Regrettably, some non-patentable therapies will never receive FDA approval because of the high cost of navigating the agency's bureaucratic labyrinth. When it comes to disease prevention, the FDA has made extraordinary efforts to censor information about proper diet and supplements that would provide guidance to consumers who want to adopt healthier lifestyles.[74]

References

1. Available at: http://www.kvue.com/shared content/ nationworld/nation/0 1 2204cccanat painkillers.40e6c22 1. html. Accessed February 27, 2004.

2. Available at: http://www.fda.gov/bbs/topics/ NEWS/2004/ NEW01 008.htm. Accessed February 27, 2004.

3. Available at: http://www.fda.gov/ohrms/ dockets/ac/02/ agenda/3882A_Draft.doc. Accessed February 27, 2004.

4. Available at: http://www.fdanews.com/ 1_1 /dailynews/ 7334-1 .html. Accessed February 27, 2004.

5. Anand BS, Romero JJ, Sanduja SK, Lichtenberger LM. Phospholipid association reduces the gastric mucosal toxicity of aspirin in human subjects. *Am J Gastroenterol.* 1999 Jul; 94(7):1818–22.

6. Blakely P, McDonald BR. Acute renal failure due to acetaminophen ingestion: a case report and review of the literature. *J Am Soc Nephrol.* 1995 Jul;6(1):48–53.

7. Bonkovsky HL, Kane RE, Jones DP, Galinsky RE, Banner B. Acute hepatic and renal toxicity from low doses of acetaminophen in

the absence of alcohol abuse or malnutrition: evidence for increased suscep tibility to drug toxicity due to cardiopul monary and renal insufficiency. *Hepatology*. 1994 May;19(5):1 141–8.

8. Clemmesen JO, Ott P, Dalhoff KP, Astrup LB, Tage-Jensen U, Poulsen HE.Recommendations for treatment of paracetamol poisoning. *Ugeskr Laegr*. 1996 Nov 25; 158(48):6892–5.

9. Conti M, Malandrino S, Magistretti MJ. Protective activity of silipide on liver damage in rodents. *Jpn J Pharmacol*. 1992 Dec;60 (4):31 5–21.

10. DeLeve LD, Kaplowitz N. Glutathione metabolism and its role in hepatotoxicity.*Pharmacol Ther*. 1991 Dec;52(3):287–305.

11. Derby LE, Jick H. Acetaminophen and renal and bladder can-cer. *Epidemiology*. 1996 Jul;7(4):358–62.

12. Dunjic BS, Axelson J, Ar'Rajab A, Larsson K, Bengmark S. Gas-troprotective capability of exogenous phosphatidylcholine in experi mentally induced chronic gastric ulcers in rats. *Scand J Gastroenterol*. 1993 Jan;28(1):89–94.

13. Gago-Dominguez M., Yuan JM, Castelao JE, Ross RK, Yu MC. Regular use of anal gesics is a risk factor for renal cell carcino ma. *Br J Cancer*. 1999 Oct;81(3):542–8.

14. Graudins A, Aaron CK, Linden CH. Overdose of extended-release acetamino phen. *N Engl J Med*. 1995 Jul 20;333(3):196.

15. Jaeschke H, Werner C, Wendel A. Disposition and hepato-protection by phosphatidyl choline liposomes in mouse liver. *Chem Biol Interact*. 1987;64(1–2):127–37.

16. Jones AL. Mechanism of action and value of N-acetylcysteine in the treatmentof early and late acetaminophen poisoning: a critical review. *J Toxicol Clin Toxicol*. 1998;36(4):277–85.

17. Kaye JA, Myers MW, Jick H. Acetaminophen and the risk of renal and bladder cancer in the general practice research data-base. *Epidemiology*. 2001 Nov; 1 2(6):690–4.

18. Kind B, Krahenbuhl S, Wyss PA, Meier-Abt PJ. Clinical-toxicological case (1). Dosage of N-acetylcysteine in acute paracetamol poisoning. *Schweiz Rundsch Med Prax*. 1996 Aug 2; 85(31–32):935–8.

19. Lieber CS. Role of oxidative stress and antioxidant therapy in alcoholic andnon-alcoholic liver diseases. *Adv Pharmacol.* 1 997;38:601–28.

20. Lieber CS. Alcohol: its metabolism and interaction with nutrients. *Annu Rev Nutr.* 2000;20:395–430.

21. McLaughlin JK, Blot WJ, Mehl ES, Fraumeni JF Jr. Relation of analgesic use to renal cancer: population-based findings. *Natl Cancer Inst Monogr.* 1985 Dec;69:217–22.

22. Mitchell T, Needham A. Over-the-counter drug is treatment for Alzheimer's. *Life Extension.* November 2000:50–5.

23. Price LM, Poklis A, Johnson DE. Fatal acetaminophen poisoning with evidence ofsubendocardial necrosis of the heart. *J Forensic Sci.* 1991 May;36(3):930–5.

24. Richie JP Jr, Lang CA, Chen TS. Acetaminophen-induced depletion of glutathione and cysteine in the aging mouse kidney. *Biochem Pharmacol.* 1992 Jul 7;44(1):129–35.

25. Siegers CP, Moller-Hartmann W. Cholestyramine as an antidote against paracetamol-induced hepato-and nephro-toxicity in the rat. *Toxicol Lett.* 1989 May;47(2):179–84.

26. Uhlig S, Wendel A. Glutathione enhancement in various mouse organs and protection by glutathione isopropyl ester against liver injury. *Biochem Pharmacol.* 1990 Jun 15;39(12):1877–81.

27. Werner C, Wendel A. Hepatic uptake and antihepatotoxic properties of vitamin E and liposomes in the mouse. *Chem Biol Interact.* 1990;75(1):83–92.

28. Zhao J, Agarwal R. Tissue distribution of silibinin, the major active constituent of silymarin, in mice and its association with enhancement of phase II enzymes: implications in cancer chemoprevention. *Carcinogenesis.* 1999 Nov;20(1 1):2101–8.

29. Available at: http://www.fda.gov/cder/drug/ analgesics/ letter.htm. Accessed February 27, 2004.

30. Available at: http://www.fda.gov/cder/drug/ analgesics/ SciencePaper. htm. Accessed February 27, 2004.

31. Available at: http://www.fda.gov/ohrms/ dockets/ac/02/ transcripts/3882T1 .htm. Accessed February 27, 2004.

32. Kaye JA, Myers MW, Jick H. Acetaminophen and the risk of renal and bladder cancer in the general practice research database. *Epidemiology*. 2001 Nov; 1 2(6):690–4.

33. Available at: http://www.kidney-cancer-symptoms.com. Accessed February 27, 2004.

34. Available at: http://www.kidney-cancer symptoms.com. Accessed February 27, 2004.

35. Piper JM, Tonascia J, Matanoski GM. Heavy phenacetin use and bladder cancer in women aged 20 to 49 years. *N Engl J Med*. 1985 Aug 1;313(5):292–5.

36. Linet MS, Chow WH, McLaughlin JK, et al. Analgesics and cancers of the renal pelvis and ureter. *Int J Cancer*. 1995 Jul 4;62 (1):15–8.

37. McCredie M, Stewart JH, Day NE. Different roles for phenacetin and paracetamol in cancer of the kidney and renal pelvis. *Int J Cancer*. 1993 Jan 21 ;53(2):245–9.

38. Brunner FP, Selwood NH. End-stage renal failure due to analgesic nephropathy, its changing pattern and cardiovascular mortality. EDTA-ERA Registry Committee. *Nephrol Dial Transplant*. 1994;9(10):1371–6.

39. Stewart JH, Hobbs JB, McCredie MR. Morphologic evidence that analgesic-induced kidney pathology contributes to the progression of tumors of the renal pelvis. *Cancer*. 1999 Oct 15;86(8):1576–82.

40. Dubach UC, Rosner B, Pfister E. Epidemiologic study of abuse of analgesics containing phenacetin. Renal morbidity and mortality (1968–1979). *N Engl J Med*. 1983 Feb 17;308(7):357–62.

41. Rathbun WB, Killen CE, Holleschau AM, Nagasawa HT. Maintenance of hepatic glutathione homeostasis and prevention of acetaminophen-induced cataract in mice by L-cysteine prodrugs. *Biochem Pharmacol*. 1996 May 3;51(9):1111–6.

42. Rathbun WB, Holleschau AM, Cohen JF, Nagasawa HT. Prevention of acetaminophen and naphthalene-induced cataract and glutathione loss by CySSME. *Invest Ophthalmol Vis Sci*. 1996 Apr;37(5):923–9.

262 ■ Pharmocracy

43. Nagasawa HT, Shoeman DW, Cohen JF, Rathbun WB. Protection against acetaminophen-induced hepatotoxicity by L-CyS-SME and its N-acetyl and ethyl ester derivatives. *J Biochem Toxicol*. 1996;1 1(6):289–95.

44. Zhao C, Shichi H. Prevention of acetaminophen-induced cataract by a combination of diallyl disulfide and N-acetylcysteine. *J Ocul Pharmacol Ther*. 1998 Aug;14(4):345–55.

45. Qian W, Shichi H. Cataract formation by a semiquinone metabolite of acetaminophen in mice: possible involvement of Ca(2+) and calpain activation. *Exp Eye Res*. 2000 Dec;71(6):567–74.

46. Qian W, Shichi H. Acetaminophen produces cataract in DBA2 mice by Ah receptor-independent induction of CYP1A2. *J Ocul Pharmacol Ther*. 2000 Aug;16(4):337–44.

47. Available at: http://www.alz.org/AboutAD/ Statistics.asp. Accessed February 27, 2004.

48. Ditzler K. Efficacy and tolerability of memantine in patients with dementia syndrome. A double-blind, placebo controlled trial. *Arzneimittelforschung*. 1991 Aug;41(8):773–80.

49. Available at: http://www.lef.org/magazine/ mag2001/ july2001_awsi.html. Accessed February 27, 2004.

50. Ambrozi L, Danielczyk W. Treatment of impaired cerebral function in psychogeriatric patients with memantine—results of a phase II double-blind study. *Pharmacopsychiatry*. 1988 May;2 1(3): 144–6.

51. Wilcock G, Mobius HJ, Stoffler A; MMM 500 group. A double-blind, placebo-controlled multicentre study of memantine in mild to moderate vascular dementia (MMM500). *Int Clin Psychopharmacol*. 2002 Nov;17(6):297–305.

52. Ferris SH. Evaluation of memantine for the treatment of Alzheimer's disease. *Expert Opin Pharmacother*. 2003 Dec;4 (1 2):2305–1 3.

53. Tariot PN, Farlow MR, Grossberg GT, et al. Memantine treatment in patients with moderate to severe Alzheimer's disease already receiving donepezil: a randomized controlled trial. *JAMA*. 2004 Jan 21;291(3):317–24.

54. Available at: http://www.lef.org/magazine/ mag2001/ july2001_report_brain_01 .html. Accessed February 27, 2004.

55. Available at: http://www.fda.gov/cder/ogd/ RLD/rld_labeling_ approved_June_2001 .html. Accessed February 27, 2004.

56. Available at: http://www.fda.gov/cder/foi/appletter/2001/20 690s16ltr.pdf. Accessed February 27, 2004.

57. Available at: http://www.pbs.org/wgbh/ pages/frontline/ shows/prescription/. Accessed February 27, 2004.

58. Available at: http://www.commondreams.org/ pressreleases/ Dec98/120298c.htm. Accessed February 27, 2004.

59. Available at: http: //www.cato.org/dailys/1-29–97.html. Accessed February 27, 2004.

60. Available at: http://www.pbs.org/wgbh/ pages/frontline/ shows/prescription/hazard/. Accessed February 27, 2004.

61. Available at: http://www.lef.org/magazine/ mag2001/ june2001_report_fda.html. Accessed February 27, 2004.

62. Available at: http://www.lef.org/magazine/ mag2000/ sep2000_report_rezulin.html. Accessed February 27, 2004.

63. Available at: http://www.life-enhancement.com/ article_template.asp?ID=206. Accessed February 27, 2004.

64. Available at: http://www.lef.org/magazine/ mag2002/ jul2002_awsi_01 .html. Accessed February 27, 2004.

65. Available at: http://www.lef.org/magazine/ mag2003/ mar2003_cover_effects_02.html. Accessed February 27, 2004.

66. Available at: http://www.lef.org/magazine/ mag2000/ dec2000_awsi.html. Accessed February 27, 2004.

67. Available at: http://www.newmediaexplorer.org/ chris/2003/07/22/access_to_medical_treatment_act_amta. htm. Accessed February 27, 2004.

68. Available at: http://www.newmediaexplorer.org/chris/control_ tactics.htm. Accessed February 27, 2004.

69. Available at: http://www.lef.org/magazine/mag2001/ sep2001 _awsi.html. Accessed February 27, 2004.

70. Available at: http://www.lef.org/magazine/ mag2001/ july2001_awsi.html. Accessed February 27, 2004.

71. Available at: http://www.lef.org/featured-articles/track2. html. Accessed February 27, 2004.

72. Available at: http://www.lef.org/magazine/ mag2001/ feb2001_awsi.html. Accessed February 27, 2004.

73. Available at: http://www.lef.org/magazine/mag99/ may99-cover.html. Accessed February 27, 2004.

74. Available at: http://tobaccodocuments.org/pm/ 2046936740–6743.html. Accessed February 27, 2004.

Dangerous Medicine

THE FDA CLAIMS that the drugs it approves are "safe." This charade is rapidly collapsing. PBS television's investigative series *Frontline* has aired a shocking exposé of dangerous prescription drugs and the FDA's complicity in allowing this outrage to occur.[1]

The *Frontline* producers initially investigated drugs that had been withdrawn from the market. After filming began, current and former FDA employees started coming forward to give a powerful critique of what really goes on inside the agency. As the story evolved, rather than making a documentary about drug safety, *Frontline* ended up shifting its focus to the FDA itself.

A major emphasis of the documentary was the FDA's reliance on drug companies' research of their own products to determine safety. As *Frontline* found out, the FDA does not conduct clinical trials, because the agency is not in the business of conducting medical research. The FDA instead reviews the results submitted by pharmaceutical companies. This means that the basis for FDA approval of a new drug is often "safety data" provided by the very company that makes the drug!

Frontline exposed this questionable drug approval sham to the world in a one-hour broadcast aired November 17, 2003. It was FDA drug reviewers who made the most appalling disclosures. These current and former FDA employees revealed incidences in which drug dangers were clearly present but were ignored or covered up by higher-level FDA officials. Only after many injuries and deaths were these drugs withdrawn or relabeled. A survey of all FDA employees showed a significant number felt they were pressured by others in the agency to give favorable reviews to dangerous and ineffective drugs.

The most absurd part of this saga is the FDA's historical record of attempting to restrict consumers' access to dietary supplements. The FDA deceitfully implies that supplements have hidden dangers. Yet the data supporting the safety and efficacy of nutrients usually come from independent sources, as opposed to the company-sponsored studies the FDA relies on to certify drug safety.

Frontline showed that in too many cases, the safety data supplied by drug companies are flawed and altered, with the result being an alarming number of injuries and deaths from prescription drug toxicities. Deaths from adverse drug reactions have become so commonplace that they rarely make the news.

For the past 18 years, *Life Extension*® has harshly criticized this corrupt system of drug approval. What *Life Extension*® lacked was the "inside" data gathered by *Frontline* that show specifically how the FDA conspires with the drug industry to approve dangerous drugs. Even more disturbing are instances in which the FDA allows toxic drugs to remain on the market even after injuries and deaths are reported. If the FDA had even a vestige of credibility remaining about its role of "protecting" the public against dangerous drugs, this *Frontline* documentary tore it to shreds. The emperor (the FDA) clearly has no clothes (credibility).

DRUGS OFTEN DO NOT WORK

In a stunning admission, a senior executive with Britain's largest pharmaceutical company has stated that most prescription medicines do not work on half the patients who take them.

Dr. Allen Roses is worldwide vice-president of genetics at GlaxoSmithKline. He is a world-class pioneer in the branch of medicine that studies the relationship between our genes and our response to individual drugs. On December 8, 2003, a British newspaper quoted Dr. Roses telling a scientific conference in London: "The vast majority of drugs only work in 30 or 50% of the people."[2]

Dr. Roses predicted that in a few years, scientists would be able to give patients a simple genetics test that would predict which medicines would work for them. Drug companies could use the information to tailor new drugs aimed at the 50% of people not helped.

It is an open secret within the pharmaceutical industry that most of its products are ineffective in most patients, but this is the first time that such a senior drug boss has gone public. Dr. Roses' admission corroborates what FDA reviewers told *Frontline*—not only are many dangerous drugs wrongfully approved, but they often are only minimally effective!

GOVERNMENT-PROTECTED MEDICINE
IS DANGEROUS MEDICINE

The word regulate can be defined as "to control or direct according to rule, principle, or law."[3]

In the US, all aspects of medical care are heavily "regulated" by the government. The end result is that healthcare is expensive, complicated, dangerous, and often ineffective.

The only way out of this bureaucratic abyss is serious free-market reform. This will not happen as long as the public thinks it needs government "protection." The producers of *Frontline* exposed the fact that the FDA does not protect Americans against unsafe drugs. Soon after the *Frontline* program aired, the most popular news program in the US contacted Life Extension® seeking information about problems with prescription drugs. It appears that the mainstream media may finally be targeting the FDA.

UPDATE

FDA's many failures have been widely reported in the media, but Congress has done nothing to change the law in a meaningful way.

References

1. Dangerous prescription [transcript]. *"Frontline."* PBS television. November 17, 2003.
2. Glaxo chief: our drugs do not work on most patients. *The Independent*. December 8, 2003.
3. Available at: http://www.dictionary.com/. Accessed December 31, 2003.

2003

Patient Advocates Sue FDA Over Drug Access

I T TAKES THE FOOD AND DRUG ADMINISTRATION an average of nearly seven years to approve promising new anti-cancer drugs. For most terminally ill patients, that's not nearly fast enough. Now patient advocates are taking the FDA to court in an effort to force the agency to streamline its approval process.

In late July, the Washington Legal Foundation sued the FDA and the Department of Health and Human Services in US District Court on behalf of the Abigail Alliance for Better Access to Developmental Drugs, a Virginia-based advocacy group for terminally ill patients. The lawsuit contends that the FDA's tortuous drug-approval process effectively denies terminally ill cancer patients access to experimental anti-cancer drugs, thereby violating their constitutional rights.

Alliance founder Frank Burroughs named the group after his daughter Abigail, who two years ago succumbed to cancer at age 21 after trying unsuccessfully to obtain access to two experimental anti-cancer drugs. The group's lawsuit also details the struggles faced by other Alliance patients who were urged by their physicians to try experimental drugs after traditional therapies failed. None of the Alliance patients was able to get into the very limited group who participated in the drug companies' clinical trials.

The lawsuit calls on the FDA to give special initial approval to experimental drugs that show effectiveness and to permit their sale and distribution to patients with no other approved treatment options. The FDA was withholding comment pending review of the lawsuit.

UPDATE

Despite several lawsuits filed against the FDA seeking early access to experimental drugs, the agency still retains dictatorial power that results in needless suffering and death of millions of Americans each year.

2002

The FDA Versus the American Consumer

S INCE 1984, THE LIFE EXTENSION FOUNDATION® has battled against the high-cost of prescription drugs. We long ago predicted that a healthcare cost crisis would erupt if Congress did not reign in the artificially inflated prices that Americans pay for their prescription medications.

To expose the incestuous relationship that exists between the FDA and the pharmaceutical giants, we made hundreds of appearances on TV and radio shows, mailed out millions of pieces of mail, ran full-page newspaper ads and set up anti-FDA web sites. We did this for the purpose of encouraging consumers to act-up against blatant corruption that is bankrupting the nation's healthcare system.

Some people ask why our scientific organization, whose mission is to discover novel methods of preventing disease and controlling aging, is so concerned about prescription drug costs. The most compelling reason is that seriously ill people join the Life Extension Foundation® seeking our medical expertise. Far too often, the elaborate drug cocktails we recommend to combat their disease are cost-prohibitive. Insurance companies frequently refuse to pay for our drug recommendations because the FDA does not officially sanction them. While the individual drugs we recommend may be FDA-approved, the agency does not recognize the off-label benefits these drugs can provide. Insurance companies then use the FDA's non-recognition as an excuse to deny coverage.[1]

The end result is that human beings are needlessly dying because of bureaucratic red tape that delays and denies them access to lifesaving medications.[2-4]

LIFE ACROSS THE BORDER

There is no inherent reason why prescription drugs cost so much. The identical medications can be purchased in Europe and Canada at far lower prices.[5] This price gouging has gone on since as early as 1959.[6] The trouble is that the FDA has attempted to deceive Congress into believing that drugs from other countries are counterfeit or contaminated. Life Extension® has shown that the FDA's assertions are baseless, false and misleading.[7]

On June 7, 2001, the FDA told Congress that they wanted to halt almost all small shipments of foreign drugs mailed to consumers in the US.[8] The only exemption would be for compassionate use, so that seriously ill patients who have exhausted all approved treatments could order drugs from overseas. The FDA told Congress: "We need to be able to make a blanket assessment that these things are not safe for American consumers and should be turned back."

In response to the FDA's assertions, Life Extension® sent Freedom of Information Act (FOIA) requests in June 2001 asking the FDA to substantiate their sworn testimony before Congress that drugs imported from other countries were dangerous.

Even though the FDA is legally mandated to respond to Freedom of Information Act requests, they have ignored our repeated written requests and phone calls to substantiate their sworn testimony about the supposed dangers of imported medications.

In 1991, Life Extension® sued the FDA for failing to respond to Freedom of Information Act (FOIA) requests dealing with this same issue. The FDA capitulated on this lawsuit and had to turn over embarrassing records to Life Extension®. Despite the FDA being forced to turn over documents to Life Extension® in 1991, the FDA continues to ignore our legitimate requests to substantiate sworn testimony made to Congress that imported drugs are dangerous.

BATTLING THE DRUG CARTEL

When the FDA told Congress that drugs imported from other countries are not safe, they provided no evidence to substantiate this intimidating allegation. The fact that no one asked the FDA to validate their baseless assertion is an indication of official apathy and the effects of massive influence peddling by pharmaceutical giants.

Life Extension® has meticulously exposed the charade of prescription drug pricing. Drug price comparison charts published in *Life Extension Magazine*® have been enlarged for presentation on the House floor to show Representatives how much more Americans pay for prescription drugs compared to Canadians and Europeans.

Despite lobbying efforts by the pharmaceutical industry, the Senate passed a bill by a vote of 69 to 30 on July 17, 2002 that would allow licensed pharmacists and drug wholesalers to import drugs that have been approved by the FDA from Canada.[9]

Large pharmaceutical companies are determined to use their political influence to block passage of this bill in the House of Representatives. The *New York Times* reports that even if a drug importation bill is passed, the Bush Administration will refuse to carry out the provisions, thereby denying Americans access to lower cost medications.[10] In December 2000, the Clinton Administration blocked implementation of a similar bill passed by the House and Senate that permitted Americans to import lower cost medications from other countries.

A battle is being waged against a drug cartel that is determined to protect its monopoly. Drug companies work hand-in-hand with the FDA to force Americans to pay the highest prices in the world for their medications.

THE DEBATE IN CONGRESS RAGES ON

The number one issue before Congress today is the high cost of prescription drugs. Consumers have besieged Congress with complaints that drugs their doctors say are necessary to keep them alive are unaffordable.

Several bills were debated this summer in Congress that would appropriate tax dollars to subsidize prescription drug programs. The problem is that the cost of drugs has become so enormous, that even the Federal government cannot figure out how to fund the gargantuan expense. The debate involved spending between 370 and 564 billion tax dollars over the next 10 years on drug subsidies. These proposals would not solve the problem, but do shift some of the burden from consumers to taxpayers.

Since most drug consumers are also taxpayers, Congress was essentially proposing to take more tax dollars from American citizens in order to subsidize the artificially inflated prices of their prescription drugs. That means that the true beneficiary of the bills debated in Congress would have been the drug industry, which would have pocketed enormous profits directly from consumers, insurance companies and the Federal government.

Another problem with tax dollars being used to pay for prescription drugs is the inevitable waste, mismanagement and fraud that occurs when government bureaucracies try to regulate the marketplace. The Federal government has had to litigate against large drug companies after finding that Medicare and Medicaid sharply overpaid for dozens of drugs. Government officials have sought billions of dollars in restitution based on their contention that drug companies induced Medicare and Medicaid to pay inflated prices for prescription medications.

In election years, everyone in Congress tries to show their constituents that they want to make prescription drugs affordable. The problem is that it is impossible to circumvent the catastrophic effects that the current FDA-protected drug monopoly creates. In the first place, there are no surplus tax dollars available to fund these proposed programs, meaning the government will go deeper into debt to fund them. Secondly, the proposed bills would not have sufficiently lowered the price of prescription drugs to the consumer.

By July 31, 2002, Congress rejected the proposed drug subsidy bills and the issue is not expected to be raised before the elections.

UPDATE

Unfortunately, just a year later, pharmaceutical lobbyists persuaded Congress to enact the Medicare Prescription

Drug Act (described in the Preamble of this book) that may force taxpayers to subsidize over 1 trillion in artificially inflated prescription drug costs.

COMPARISON OF US, EUROPEAN, AND CANADIAN DRUG PRICES

Drug	Qty	Potency	US Price	European Price	Canadian Price
Augmentin®	12	500 mg	$55.50	$8.75	$12.00
Cipro®	20	500 mg	$87.99	$40.75	$53.55
Claritin®	30	10 mg	$89.00	$18.75	$37.50
Coumadin®	100	5 mg	$64.88	$15.80	$24.94
Glucophage®	100	850 mg	$124.65	$22.00	$26.47
Norvasc®	30	10 mg	$67.00	$33.00	$46.27
Paxil®	30	20 mg	$83.29	$49.00	$44.35
Pravachol®	28	10 mg	$85.60	$29.00	$40.00
Premarin®	100	0.625 mg	$55.42	$8.95	$22.46
Prempro®	28	0.625 mg	$31.09	$5.75	$14.33
Prilosec®	30	20 mg	$112.00	$49.25	$59.00
Prozac®	20	20 mg	$91.08	$18.50	$20.91
Synthroid®	100	0.1 mg	$33.93	$8.50	$13.22
Zestril®	28	20 mg	$40.49	$20.00	$20.44
Zocor®	28	10 mg	$123.43	$28.00	$45.49
Zoloft®	30	100 mg	$114.56	$52.50	$47.40

This chart and the chart on page 284 were compiled during different time periods. That is why the price of some of the drugs varies between the two charts.

A REAL SOLUTION TO THE HEALTHCARE COST CRISIS

Congressman Gil Gutknecht of Minnesota has written an amendment to a Medicare bill that prohibits the FDA from blocking importation by individuals and pharmacies of FDA-approved drugs. If this amendment is passed, it will help solve the prescription drug crisis without the need for taxpayer subsidies.

Two years ago, Congress passed legislation to allow Americans to import wholesale quantities of lower-cost prescription drugs into the United States. But the promise of this legislation has gone unfulfilled. Even though the FDA largely wrote the bill, and Congress provided the $23 million the FDA requested to implement the bill, then-Secretary Shalala refused to implement the measure. The result? Drug prices in Europe and elsewhere are still 30% to 300% lower than in the United States. Prices have not equalized. Americans still pay the highest prices in the world to subsidize the "starving Swiss." Even former Secretary Shalala admits this fact.

But that's not all. The FDA refuses not only to allow wholesale importation, the FDA also maintains that personal importation is illegal. Yet, because the market for lower-cost drugs is so large, the FDA looks the other way when people import personal-use quantities of prescription drugs. That's right: the FDA today allows folks to carry drugs over the border, and apparently now even allows [them] to mail order drugs from abroad. Yet all the while, the FDA publicly maintains such importation is illegal, thus threatening importers with dire legal consequences.

This is wrong. The FDA can't have it both ways. Either personal use importation is illegal, or it's not. Last year, by a vote of 324 to 101, the House passed language explicitly allowing individual Americans to import lower-cost FDA-approved drugs from FDA-approved facilities. This is common sense, and it is the FDA's current policy.

Unfortunately the Senate refused to pass this amendment, so the FDA continues to hold a legal dagger over the heads of those who try to import FDA-approved drugs.

Fortunately, with the House drug coverage bill coming to the floor soon, we have an opportunity to codify current FDA practice, AND allow our nation's pharmacists to offer the same drugs. With this, all Americans can be sure they have the right to save money on their prescription drugs.

The Congressional Budget Office estimates prescription drugs will cost Medicare beneficiaries $1.8 trillion over the next 10 years. Americans could save $630 billion from this bill if they could be allowed access to the same drugs from FDA-approved facilities throughout the world.[11] Price, not coverage, is the real prescription drug problem. The FDA should not stand between American consumers and lower drug prices. The Gutknecht Amendment (H.R. 5186) prohibits the FDA from blocking importation by individuals and pharmacies of FDA-approved prescription drugs from FDA-approved facilities.[12]

THE SHOCKING TRUTH BEHIND PRESCRIPTION DRUG PRICES

Do you ever wonder how much it costs a drug company to obtain the active ingredient in a prescription medication? Life Extension® did a search of offshore chemical synthesizers that supply the active ingredients found in drugs approved by the FDA.

A significant percentage of drugs sold in the United States contain active ingredients that are actually synthesized in other countries. Drug companies import these active ingredients into the United States where they wind up in the expensive drugs you buy at the local pharmacy. While the FDA says you cannot trust drugs from other countries, the facts are that most of the drugs sold in the United States contain active ingredients synthesized in the very countries the FDA says you cannot trust.

In our independent investigation of how much profit drug companies really make, we obtained the actual price of active ingredients used in some of the most popular drugs sold in America.

The astounding profit margin enjoyed by drug companies exposes several facts. First, it shows why the pharmaceutical industry is the most profitable of all businesses. But since large drug companies only make around 15% net profit margins, it also exposes the incredible cost drug companies bear to comply with today's burdensome drug approval system.* If the FDA relaxed its drug approval standards, the cost of bringing new patented drugs could be reduced.

These exorbitant profit margins also provide incentive for drug companies to get their patented molecules approved by the FDA, whether they kill people or not. Horror stories abound of how drug companies have egregiously falsified data to obtain FDA approval.†

Many consumers are nervous about the FDA becoming less stringent, but the facts are that today's regulatory system is allowing lethal drugs on the marketplace and also acting as a disincentive for drug companies to develop novel drugs to save lives.

Take the cholesterol-lowering drug Baycol®, for example, which was removed from the market after killing 100 people.‡ Baycol® is a statin drug that works via a mechanism similar to that in Mevacor®, Zocor®, Lipitor®, Pravachol®, etc. Was there a need for tens of millions of dollars to be spent developing another statin drug? Drug companies think so, because the FDA readily recognizes statin drugs, so they are easy to get approved.

---

* Stephen S. Hall, "Claritin and Schering-Plough: A Prescription for Profit." http://senrs. com/a_prescription_for_profit.htm

† David Willman, "The Rise and Fall of the Killer Drug Rezulin," *Life Extension Magazine*®, September 2000.

‡ "More deaths linked to Bayer's Lipobay," January 18, 2002. http://news.ft.com/ft/ gx.cgi/ftc?pagename=View&c=Article&cid=FT3HZ3AFMWC &live=true&tagid=IX LHT5GTICC&subheading=heal

The problem is that no life was saved because of Baycol®. Anyone who may have benefitted from Baycol® could have obtained the same results from other statin drugs. So when drug companies justify the high price of drugs because of research costs, remember that most of the so-called novel compounds they develop will not save a single life, as they are no different than what is already available.

WHAT DRUGS REALLY COST

Brand Name	Consumer Price	Cost of Active Ingredient	Percent Markup
Celebrex® 100 mg	$130.27	$0.60	21,712%
Claritin® 10 mg	$215.17	$0.71	30,306%
Keflex® 250 mg	$157.39	$1.88	8,372%
Lipitor® 20 mg	$272.37	$5.80	4,696%
Norvasc® 10 mg	$188.29	$0.14	134,493%
Paxil® 20 mg	$220.27	$7.60	2,898%
Prevacid® 30 mg	$344.77	$1.01	34,136%
Prilosec® 20 mg	$360.97	$0.52	69,417%
Prozac® 20 mg	$247.47	$0.11	224,973%
Tenormin® 50 mg	$104.47	$0.13	80,362%
Vasotec® 10 mg	$102.37	$0.20	51,185%
Xanax® 1 mg	$136.79	$0.024	569,958%
Zestril® 20 mg	$89.89	$3.20	2,809%
Zithromax® 600 mg	$1,482.19	$18.78	7,892%
Zocor® 40 mg	$350.27	$8.63	4,059%
Zoloft® 50 mg	$206.87	$1.75	11,821%

Now that you know the outrageous profit margins on prescription drugs, you can understand why drug companies do almost anything to prevent competition from developing. Large drug companies intensely lobby Congress to pass laws that give them extra time of exclusivity, file lawsuits to delay generic competition, petition the FDA to stop the importation of lower cost medications, and go as far as to pay off generic companies to not compete.

Drug companies spend big dollars protecting their illicit monopoly, all of which is reflected in the price consumers pay for their prescription drugs.

BREAKING THE DRUG MONOPOLY

The Gutknecht Amendment provides Americans access to FDA-approved prescription drugs made in FDA-approved facilities at world market prices. Passage of this amendment could abolish high prices of prescription drugs forever.

While drugs sold in Europe and Canada do cost less than their American counterparts, they are still artificially high because of regulations in these other countries that stifle competition. If Americans are allowed to freely import prescription drugs from FDA-approved manufacturing facilities in other countries, there will be a surge of new laboratories that will seek FDA-certification. The result will be a flood of super low-cost drugs into the United States as various FDA-certified laboratories compete fiercely on quality and price.

When Congressional leaders debate the prescription drug cost crisis, few of them understand the huge discrepancy that exists between the cost of the active drug ingredient compared to the price charged for the brand name or generic drug. For instance, consumers pay $360.00 for 100 capsules of the stomach-acid suppressing drug Prilosec®. The cost of the active ingredient for 100 capsules of Prilosec®, however, is only 52 cents. There will soon be a generic version of Prilosec® available, but because of FDA overregulation, the cost per 100 capsules will probably be around $80.00. In a free market environment, where many companies could offer generic Prilosec® products instead of the chosen few anointed by the FDA, a product whose active ingredient costs 52 cents (like Prilosec®) would be available to consumers for under $7.00 a bottle.

A free market environment would eliminate the prescription drug cost crisis because the FDA would not be allowed to protect a monopoly that enables both brand name and generic companies to charge extortionist prices for lifesaving medications.

Drug company lobbyists are inundating Congress to prevent any type of prescription drug importation bill from becoming law. Consumer groups are intimidated by the FDA's baseless assertions that imported drugs are somehow dangerous. The FDA has preyed on fear and uncertainty for decades, while American consumers are extorted into paying the highest prices in the world for their prescription drugs.

This is not just an issue for individuals to be concerned with. There are dire predictions of severe economic upheavals in the United States if a solution is not found for the high cost of prescription drugs. Some of the largest corporations in America cannot afford to fund health insurance benefits for current and retired employees. Health insurance companies are going bankrupt because of astronomical drug prices. Medicare itself is facing insolvency.

The United States has been economically deteriorating as prescription drug prices skyrocket. In order to counter the influence peddling of the pharmaceutical behemoths, American consumers must become politically active. Consumers vastly outnumber drug industry lobbyists. Regrettably, ignorance and apathy have silenced many Americans and enabled drug money to create laws that favor outlandish pharmaceutical company profits at the expense of the consumer.

If the Gutknecht Amendment is passed, it will liberate the American consumer from becoming an economic serf to the pharmaceutical cartel.

UPDATE

The Gutknecht bill passed and was signed into law. The FDA used a technicality to nix it, which resulted in windfall profits for the pharmaceutical industry as America plummeted into fiscal crisis.

References

1. "We Need an FDA Leader, Not a Regulatory Czar Healthcare: AIDS, cancer and Alzheimer's are among the issues where David Kessler has compromised science and ethics." The *Los Angeles Times* (Pre-1997 Fulltext), Feb 10, 1993.

2. "A National Survey Of Emergency Room Physicians Regarding The Food And Drug Administration," by Gregory Conko. October 1, 1999. http://www.cei.org/gencon/025,02298.cfm

3. "A National Survey Of Neurologists And Neurosurgeons Regarding The Food And Drug Administration," by Gregory Conko. October 5, 1998. http://www.cei.org/gencon/025,01586.cfm

4. "Who Is Mary J. Ruwart?" *Life Extension Magazine®*, July 2001. http://www.lef.org/magazine/mag2001/july2001_cover_ruwart.html

5. "Claritin and Schering-Plough: A Prescription for Profit," by Stephen S. Hall. http://senrs.com/a_prescription_for_profit.htm

6. "What's New About Prescription. . .," by Morton Mintz. *Washington Post*, Page B1, February 11, 2001.

7. "Drugs The FDA Says You Can't Have," *Life Extension Magazine®*, July 2001.

8. Statement of William K. Hubbard, Senior Associate Commissioner for Policy, Planning and Legislation, Food and Drug Administration, before the Subcommittee on Oversight and Investigations Committee on Energy and Commerce, US House of Representative, June 7, 2001. http://www.fda.gov/ola/2001/drugimport0607.html

9. Greater Access to Affordable Phamacauticals Act of 2001. Senate, July 17, 2002. http://thomas.loc.gov/cgi-bin/bdquery/z?d107:H.R.1862:

10. "Thursday Plan to Import Drugs From Canada Passes In Senate, but Bush Declines to Carry It Out," by Robert Pear. Late Edition, Final, Section A, Page 14, Column 4. *New York Times* National Desk, July 18, 2002.

11. CBO Testimony, statement of Dan L. Crippen, Director Projections of Medicare and Prescription Drug Spending, before the Committee on Finance United States Senate, March 7, 2002. http://www.cbo.gov/showdoc.cfm?index=3304&sequence=0

12. Drug Importation Act of 2002 (Introduced in House), HR 5186 IH 107th Congress, 2d Session H. R. 5186, to amend the Federal Food, Drug, and Cosmetic Act with respect to the importation of prescription drugs. In the House of Representative, July 23, 2002. http://thomas.loc.gov/

Supreme Court Roundup

O
N APRIL 30, 2002, declaring that "regulating speech must be a last-not first-resort," the Supreme Court invalidated a provision of the federal food and drug laws that banned pharmacies from advertising the availability of "compounded" pharmaceuticals, drugs that pharmacists make themselves by mixing ingredients to meet the specific medical needs of certain patients.

A 1997 federal law that barred such advertising reflected federal regulators' concern that compounded drugs did not go through the detailed screening for safety and effectiveness to which drug companies have to submit their mass-produced drugs. Congress wanted to limit consumer access to compounded drugs, which protected large pharmaceutical companies from lower cost competition.

But the 5-to-4 decision on April 30th said that "the government simply has not provided sufficient justification here" for choosing a restriction on speech rather than other possible ways to restrict access to compounded drugs, which generally are not commercially available and which patients may receive only by a doctor's prescription.

"We have made clear that if the government could achieve its interests in a manner that does not restrict speech, or that restricts less speech, the government must do so," Justice Sandra Day O'Connor said for the majority.

The real debate on the court was not over drug policy but over the constitutional value to assign to commercial speech. While the majority opinion today did not break ground, it was a powerful indication that the value a majority of the court assigns to commercial speech is high and getting higher.

Justice O'Connor's majority opinion outlined alternatives that, in the court's view, Congress should have used before turning to an advertising ban, most dealing with limitations on the amount of compounded drugs an individual pharmacy could make or sell. Or the government could require warning labels advising consumers that the compounded drug had not gone through the usual approval process, Justice O'Connor said.

"The government has not offered any reason why these possibilities, alone or in combination, would be insufficient to prevent compounding from occurring on such a scale as to undermine the new drug approval process," she said, adding, "Indeed, there is no hint that the government even considered these or any other alternatives."

She continued: "If the First Amendment means anything, it means that regulating speech must be a last-not first-resort. Yet here it seems to have been the first strategy the government thought to try."

The legal status of compounded drugs after the decision today was not immediately clear. The government took the position that such drugs were not legal before the

1997 law, the Food and Drug Administration Modernization Act, which made their lawful sale contingent on the
advertising ban and on other restrictions. The Ninth Circuit, holding that the various provisions of the law could
not be considered separately, struck down the entire statute, an aspect of its ruling that the court did not address
on April 30th.

UPDATE

Compounding pharmacies later won significant legal victories against the FDA, but compounding pharmacies are
still prohibited from competing on a level playing field
against Big Pharma.

2001

Are Offshore Drugs Dangerous?

I F YOU SUFFER FROM TYPE II DIABETES, you're likely to be prescribed a drug called Glucophage®. This drug lowers glucose and other blood risk factors that cause lethal diabetic complications.

Glucophage® works by enhancing cell sensitivity to the effects of insulin. Since type II diabetes is characterized by cellular insulin resistance, the fact that Glucophage® helps restore insulin sensitivity makes it a potent weapon against a disease that currently afflicts 16 million Americans. Clinical studies dating back to the 1950s demonstrate Glucophage®'s efficacy and safety when properly used.

For several decades, Americans could not legally obtain Glucophage®. That's because the FDA said it was toxic and banned its sale in the US. The Europeans did not agree that Glucophage® posed a health risk and approved its use decades ago.*

---

* Glucophage® is the brand name for the generic drug metformin, one of the most popular anti-diabetic drugs prescribed today.

The FDA was proven wrong about Glucophage® and the drug was finally approved in December 1994. It is difficult to calculate exactly how many Americans died while Glucophage® was kept out of the United States. It is very easy, however, to document that American consumers are being price gouged because of the FDA's error. A one-month supply of Glucophage® costs $4.12 in other countries, while Americans pay $32.83 for the same quantity.

The reason for this unconscionable price disparity is that Glucophage® is old news in Europe, where it has been used since the 1960s. The FDA's delay in approval has enabled Glucophage® to enjoy a virtual monopoly in the United States, causing US citizens to pay more than seven times the price this same drug sells for in other countries.

The number of people who die each year from diabetic complications is staggering. American diabetics perished while Glucophage® was being safely used throughout the world. Because of FDA ineptitude, US citizens pay grossly inflated prices to obtain a drug (Glucophage®) that is more than 30 years old.

THE FDA'S LATEST CHARADE

The FDA now has the audacity to ask Congress to ban just about ALL imports of medications from other countries under the guise of "protecting" Americans against dangerous drugs.

On June 7, 2001, the FDA told Congress that they want to halt almost all small shipments of foreign drugs mailed to consumers in the US. The FDA wants US Custom Service agents to send back all small foreign drug shipments they find. The only exemption would be for "compassionate use," so that seriously ill patients who have exhausted all approved treatments could order drugs from overseas that are unavailable in the US.

The FDA says it needs to turn away all foreign drug shipments because of the sheer volume of drugs being imported. More American consumers are learning they can obtain prescription drugs at a fraction of the price charged in the US. The FDA now admits that the number of shipments far exceeds the agency's ability to review them on a case-by-case basis. The FDA told Congress, "We need to be able to make a blanket assessment that these things are not safe for American consumers and should be turned back."

The fraud being perpetrated by the FDA is the assertion that medications imported from other countries are automatically illegal, counterfeit or contaminated. This is what the FDA would have said about Glucophage® before they approved it in 1994. The facts are that drugs from other countries cost far less and are sometimes more advanced than what is available on the American marketplace.

The FDA told Congress that an estimated 2 million packages containing drugs enter the United States through international mail each year. "The inescapable conclusion is these drugs are virtually all unapproved in the United States. . . . They may be counterfeit or worse," the FDA said to Congress.

The truth is that most of the drugs the FDA complains about are already FDA-approved and are manufactured by the same companies that sell them to American pharmacies. The FDA is using scare tactics to protect the profits of the pharmaceutical industry . . . not the health of the public.

Currently, the law says that Customs must contact recipients if it detains drugs at the border. The FDA's new proposal would waive that requirement. In other words, the FDA wants all drugs to be turned away without even providing the US citizen (who paid for the drug) with a notice and opportunity to explain why they need them.[1]

Drugs the FDA says are safe kill over 100,000 Americans every year, while the agency cannot demonstrate drugs imported from other countries are hurting anyone.

That's not to say that some day an American won't suffer an adverse reaction from an imported drug. After all, many of the drugs being imported are the same FDA-approved medications that are killing over 100,000 Americans every year.[2-4]

The FDA denied Glucophage® to Americans for decades, but rapidly approved Rezulin® to treat Type II diabetics. Rezulin® killed about 391 Americans before it was withdrawn, according to a tabulation done by the *Los Angeles Times*.[5] Those afflicted with Type II diabetes suffered and died waiting for the FDA's belated approval of the relatively safe drug Glucophage®.*

So while the FDA brazenly testified before Congress that all drugs imported from other countries are "dangerous," the facts show the agency's assertion is blatantly false and misleading.

The FDA preys on fear and uncertainty, while American consumers are extorted into paying the highest prices in the world for their prescription drugs.

UNDOING THIS TRAVESTY

The FDA lacks the moral and scientific legitimacy to deny Americans access to medications that are approved by health ministries in other countries. The FDA's delay in approving Glucophage® is a prime example of why this agency should not be allowed to embargo drugs from other countries.

---

* Note: Glucophage® is now available in the United States under the generic name metformin. Glucophage® is not for everyone. To read safety precautions about this drug, log on to www.glucophage.com.

Bureaucratic barriers at the FDA stifle the development of novel medicines, while drug company influence enables lethal drugs (like Rezulin®) to be "approved" by the agency as safe and effective.

References

1. Statement of William K. Hubbard, Senior Associate Commissioner for Policy, Planning and Legislation, Food and Drug Administration, before the Subcommittee on Oversight and Investigations Committee on Energy and Commerce, US House of Representatives, June 7, 2001. http://www.fda.gov/ola/2001/drugimport0607.html

2. Lazarou J, et al. Incidence of adverse drug reactions in hospitalized patients: a meta-analysis of prospective studies. *JAMA* 1998 Apr 1 5;279(1 5): 1200–5.

3. Bates DW. Drugs and adverse drug reactions: how worried should we be? *JAMA* 1998 Apr 15;279(15):1216–7.

4. Cimons M. "FDA Moves to Reduce Accidental Drug Deaths." *LA Times* May 10,1999. Home Edition Section: PART A Page: A-1.

5. Willman David "Rise and Fall of the Killer Drug Rezulin," *Life Extension Magazine®*, Sept. 2000, p. 3 1–39.

Drugs the FDA Says You Can't Have

AMERICANS SUFFER AND DIE even though effective drugs to treat their diseases are approved in other countries. The public is generally aware that novel drugs are sold in Europe and Japan, but intense lobbying by the pharmaceutical industry has blocked the wide-scale availability of these better medications.

Drug companies don't want Americans to shop the world for more effective therapies. They prefer the current FDA-protected system where large companies enjoy a virtual monopoly over the American marketplace. This archaic system earns record profits for drug companies at the expense of US citizens, who pay inflated prices for the medications the FDA does allow them to have.

The FDA deceives the public and Congress into believing that drugs approved in other countries are somehow "dangerous," despite having no evidence to support this. What the FDA conveniently ignores is the fact that drugs they say are "safe" kill over 106,000 Americans every year.[1–3]

THALIDOMIDE STILL KILLS

Proponents of today's drug approval system have to go back 41 years to the thalidomide debacle to find an example of an offshore drug causing a serious side effect. Thalidomide still kills because the FDA is using this old issue as an excuse to embargo life-saving drugs that are approved by health ministries in other countries. Furthermore, these drugs have been used in other countries for years without serious side effects.

Few people remember that it was not the FDA who discovered the thalidomide problem. It was a German scientist who identified thalidomide's dreadful power to halt limb development in the early stages of pregnancy. The FDA's sole contribution to avoiding this problem in the United States was a delay by a junior FDA officer in reviewing the original application.

There is tragedy on the other side of the thalidomide ledger, too. Thalidomide has been shown to halt the proliferation of blood vessels, an effect that may help starve certain cancers and protect against blindness induced by wet macular degeneration. In 1998, the FDA finally approved thalidomide to treat a complication related to leprosy. That means that doctors can legally prescribe thalidomide to patients with other diseases. The FDA, however, has put up so many restrictions on its off-label use, that few physicians or patients are willing to fight the red tape.[4]

The rare disease the FDA approved thalidomide to treat only occurs in about 50 Americans every year. The FDA, however, says the company that makes thalidomide cannot promote its use in treating cancer and macular degeneration. Recent First Amendment losses the FDA has suffered in the courts may enable thalidomide to be advertised,[5] but that would mean the company making the drug would incur the wrath of the FDA and be subjected to retaliation against other drugs it might want to get approved.

FEARING FDA RETALIATION

The FDA has taken science out of the practice of medicine and replaced it with an incompetent and biased bureaucracy. To win FDA approval of a new drug, it takes a lot of political influence.

The committees who advise the FDA whether or not to approve a new drug are largely comprised of individuals who are beholden to the pharmaceutical giants.[6] Small biotech companies who cannot afford to put their own people on these advisory committees are at a significant disadvantage. There are FDA-staffers who appear unusually friendly to large drug companies, but find every excuse imaginable to delay the approval of novel drugs from smaller companies.[7–12]

The FDA intentionally delayed the approval of ribavirin for decades while this anti-viral drug was saving lives in just about every civilized country on earth. The company who made ribavirin committed the terrible "sin" of holding a press conference to extol the virtues of this drug before the FDA approved it. Another victim of FDA retaliation was the immune-enhancing drug isoprinosine. While isoprinosine has been prescribed by doctors throughout the world for nearly two decades, the FDA will never approve it here because the manufacturer helped promote the fact that Americans could import it from other countries for their own personal use. The sad fact is that when effective drugs are not approved because of FDA retaliation, American citizens die.[13, 14]

The FDA has put up so many restrictions on its off-label use, that few physicians or patients are willing to fight the red tape.

LIFE-SAVING OFFSHORE DRUGS

An example of a drug that may never be approved in the United States is thymosin alpha-1, which is an immune boosting agent produced in the thymus gland.[15] Unfortunately, the small company making the drug lacked the resources to win FDA approval. Thymosin alpha-1 did gain approval in Europe. Published studies show that when used in combination with cancer chemotherapy, it helps mitigate bone marrow toxicity.[16, 17] When thymosin alpha-1 is combined with interleukin-2 or alpha interferon, it enhances immune response against cancer cells and the hepatitis C virus.[18-23] Thymosin alpha-1 should be available to Americans, but the FDA says no!

Another drug that could be of benefit to hepatitis C and certain cancer patients is polaprezinc. This ultra-safe Japanese drug has been shown to reduce viral load and induce complete response in Type 1b hepatitis C (when combined with interferon).[24] It may also be effective as an adjuvant therapy in cancer cells that up-regulate a growth factor called nuclear factor kappa beta. If you don't live in Japan, it is very difficult to obtain polaprezinc, a unique compound of carnosine and zinc.

Neurodegenerative diseases such as Alzheimer's have no effective treatment. A drug called memantine may delay the progression of Alzheimer's and Parkinson's disease. Memantine works by a different mechanism than current FDA-approved drugs such as Aricept® and tacrine. Memantine has been used in Germany for the last ten years, but it remains bogged down in FDA-mandated clinical trials. Four million American Alzheimer's disease patients anxiously await.[25-33]

IT'S TIME TO REVOLT

Today's flawed system of drug approval needs a major overhaul or Americans will continue to perish while effective therapies exist in other countries. As more Americans learn that they are not getting the best that science has to offer, we believe the citizenry will rebel against the medical establishment, who place their monopolistic profits ahead over the wellbeing of the patient.

The world is rapidly changing and information about non-FDA approved therapies can easily be found on the Internet. The problem for consumers is separating real science from charlatans who prey on those seeking a solution for a serious medical problem.

WHERE ARE THE BEST DRUGS?

The most advanced drugs in the world are right here in the United States, but remain bogged down in the FDA's approval quagmire. The profit potential in the American marketplace is so large that drug companies are not seeking quick approval in other countries as much as they used to.

Pharmaceutical companies spend gargantuan sums of money on clinical trials before they can earn a penny on the sale of the drug. The inordinate delay created by the FDA not only causes the needless death of those in desperate need, but it makes the cost of drugs astronomical once they finally get approved.

A better approach would be to allow pharmaceutical companies to sell new drugs before they are officially "approved." This change would result in a renaissance of new medications becoming available at far lower prices. Those doctors and people who desire FDA protection could use only FDA-approved drugs, while individuals who think the FDA moves too slowly could gain immediate access to medications they believe could help them. Wouldn't it be wonderful if nonprofit groups competed to provide unbiased advice about unapproved drugs that could save lives?

Some argue that the FDA approves new drugs too fast and should mandate more stringent testing. The facts are that the dangerous drugs the FDA approves are often the result of drug company manipulation of the already-flawed approval process.

Those who think they need the FDA forget that scientists established the efficacy of vaccines, antiseptics and antibiotics long before lawyers arrived to supervise their work. Medical science does not require the Federal government's rules or approvals to know whether a drug works. The superimposed political layer of review on research has been the major roadblock that prevents scientists from finding real cures for diseases that have too long plagued modern man.

Some pessimists are concerned that unethical companies would sell dangerous drugs in an unregulated environment, yet no private company prospers for long selling products that kill, maim or injure in an era when trial lawyers abound.

The following is an excerpt from the *Wall Street Journal* of an editorial entitled "FDA Caution Can Be Deadly, Too":

> Most ordinary, healthy people probably still take some comfort in the thought that a diligent, generally competent, well-meaning federal agency is keeping an eye on the contents of

their medicine cabinets. But we live in an age of enormously rapid progress in medical science. Impelled by genetic science, we are progressing toward ever more individualized, customized therapies. Some therapies already depend on extracting, modifying and cultivating cells, tissues or organs from the patient's own body, or from close relatives. General-issue tailoring of your medicines is fine if you happen to stand smack in the statistical middle of everything, but few real people do. And in the direst circumstances, the best therapies will often be the ones on the edges of science, well outside the bounds of the truths that have been fully certified in Washington.[34]

EDITOR OF *THE LANCET* SAYS THE FDA IS FAR TOO COZY WITH DRUG INDUSTRY

According to a May 19, 2001 editorial published in *The Lancet*, patients taking a controversial new drug for irritable bowel syndrome may have died because the FDA has become a "servant of [the drug] industry."

This devastating editorial reveals that although Glaxo-Smith Kline voluntarily withdrew the drug Lotronex® from the US market last November after the deaths of five patients, senior FDA officials are now seeking to reintroduce it.

This editorial goes on to say:

This story reveals not only dangerous failings in a single drug's approval and review process but also the extent to which the FDA, its Center for Drug Evaluation and Research (CDER) in particular, has become the servant of industry.

This two-page editorial is entitled "Lotronex® and the FDA: A Fatal Erosion of Integrity." It accuses the FDA of receiving hundreds of millions of dollars in funding from industry.

The editorial claims the views of FDA scientists who raised safety questions about the drug were dismissed by FDA officials and that these scientists were excluded from further discussion about the drug's future. It goes on to allege that negotiations between the FDA and the Glaxo on the drug's future involved a "two-track process, one official and transparent, one unofficial and covert."

The FDA approved Lotronex® in February 2000 but it was never approved by the European Medicines Evaluation Agency. The company withdrew the product in the United States in November 2000 after 49 cases of ischaemic colitis and 21 of severe constipation, including instances of obstructed and ruptured bowel. In addition to five deaths, 34 patients had required admission to hospital and 10 needed surgery.

The Lancet says that as early as July 2000, it was known that seven patients had developed serious complications. The clinical data confirmed "substantial and potentially life-threatening risks." Instead of withdrawing Lotronex®, the FDA issued a medication guide. "This decision was to prove fatal," according to *The Lancet*.

The editorial states that FDA scientists knew that the warning advising patients to stop taking Lotronex® if they felt "increasing abdominal discomfort" was impractical. The reason is that abdominal pain can be confused as a classical symptom of an irritable bowel.

FDA scientists argued that it was unreasonable to expect patients or physicians to know if this type of pain was an early warning of possibly fatal ischaemic colitis. Their view was dismissed by FDA officials. According to *The Lancet*, "The scientists who raised these issues felt intimidated by senior colleagues and were excluded from further discussions about Lotronex®'s future."

In a memorandum dated November 16, 2000, FDA scientists said, "Early warning of the dire side effects of this drug is clearly not feasible" and added a "risk management plan cannot be successful." FDA officials choose to ignore this warning.

By the time of a key November 28th, 2000 meeting between Glaxo and FDA officials, rather than reject the company's proposal to withdraw Lotronex®, the FDA offered several conciliatory options including voluntary withdrawal pending further discussion.

The Lancet claims "many within the FDA's leadership now want to bring Lotronex® back. An advisory committee meeting set up to do so is being planned for June or July."

The reason this highly critical editorial against the FDA was published is because *The Lancet* previously published some of the trial data that led to the FDA approving the drug. As increasing reports of adverse effects became known, the editor of *The Lancet* became "more intrigued about what was happening, it opened up into an issue of how science is dealt with by the FDA and how, because of industry funding, it has fatally compromised its independence."

The Lancet editor went on to say that "The scientists within the FDA who analyze and interpret adverse drug reactions have been largely ignored after the drug was approved and marketed. That is where there has been a terrible failure in evaluating the safety of this drug."

References

1. Lazarou J, et al. Incidence of adverse drug reactions in hospitalized patients: a meta-analysis of prospective studies. *JAMA* 1998 Apr 1 5;279(1 5): 1200–5.

2. Bates DW. Drugs and adverse drug reactions: how worried should we be? *JAMA* 1998 Apr 15;279(15):1216–7.

3. Cimons M. "FDA Moves to Reduce Accidental Drug Deaths." *LA Times* May 10, 1999. Home Edition Section: PART A Page: A-1.

4. Thalidomide Information. "FDA Announces Approval of Drug for Hansen's Disease (Leprosy) Side Effect—Imposes Unprecedented Authority to Restrict Distribution" http://www.fda.gov/cder/news/thalinfo/thalidomide.htm.

5. Faloon W. "What's Wrong with the FDA?—FDA Suffers Massive Defeats." May 2001 issue *Life Extension Magazine®*.

6. Cauchon Dennis. "FDA advisers tied to industry." *USA Today*; Arlington, Va.; Sep 25, 2000.

7. William David. "Scientists Who Judged Pill Safety Received Fees." *LA Times*, October 29, 1999. PART A Section.

8. William David. "2nd NIH Researcher to Become Part of Conflict Probe." *LA Times*, September 4, 1999. Home Edition PART A Section.

9. William David. "Researcher's Fees Point to Other Potential Conflicts at NIH."

10. "Deadly Medicine" by Thomas J. Moore.

11. A Letter from Roderic Dale, PhD May 2000 issue *Life Extension Magazine®*.

12. Driscoll J.P. "Perspective on Drug Policy—FDA's 'Caution' Is Killing People; Unnecessary delays in approval for vital drugs and medical devices are more dangerous than thalidomide." *LA Times*, June 4, 1995. Home Edition Section: Opinion Piece Page: M-5.

13. FDA vs ICN Pharmaceuticals, Drug: Ribavirin.

14. FDA versus Newport Pharmaceuticals, Drug: Isoprinsoine.

15. Anti-Aging News Vol. 1 No. 11 November 1981 "Thymosin: The Immunity Hormone."

16. Ohta Y, et al. Thymosin alpha 1 exerts protective effect against the 5-FU induced bone marrow toxicity. *Int J Immunopharmacol* 1 985;7(5):761–8.

17. Ohta Y, et al. Immunomodulating activity of thymosin fraction 5 and thymosin alpha 1 in immunosuppressed mice. *Cancer Immunol Immunother* 1983; 15(2): 108–13.

18. Moscarella S, et al. Interferon and thymosin combination therapy in naive patients with chronic hepatitis C: preliminary results. *Liver* 1998 Oct;18(5):366–9.

19. Sherman KE, et al. Combination therapy with thymosin alpha1 and interferon for the treatment of chronic hepatitis C infection: a randomized, placebo-controlled double-blind trial. *Hepatology* 1998 Apr;27(4):1 128–35.

20. Garaci E, et al. Thymosin alpha 1 in the treatment of cancer: from basic research to clinical application. *Int J Immunopharmacol* 2000 Dec;22(1 2): 1067–76.

21. Beuth J, et al. Thymosin alpha(1) application augments immune response and down-regulates tumor weight and organ colonization in BALB/c-mice. *Cancer Lett* 2000 Oct 16;159(1):9–13.

22. Moody TW, et al. Thymosinalpha1 is chemopreventive for lung adenoma formation in A/J mice. *Cancer Lett* 2000 Jul 31;155 (2):121–7.

23. Pica F, et al. High doses of Thymosin alpha 1 enhance the anti-tumor efficacy of combination chemo-immunotherapy for murine B 16 melanoma. *Anticancer Res* 1998 Sep-Oct; 1 8(5A):3571–8.

24. Nagamine T, et al. Preliminary study of combination therapy with interferon-alpha and zinc in chronic hepatitis C patients with genotype 1b. *Biol Trace Elem Res* 2000 Summer;75(1–3):53–63.

25. Winblad B, et al. Memantine in severe dementia: results of the 9M-Best Study (Benefit and efficacy in severely demented patients during treatment with memantine). *Int J Geriatr Psychiatry* 1999 Feb;14(2):135–46.

26. Schneider E, et al. [Effects of oral memantine administration on Parkinson symptoms. Results of a placebo-controlled multicenter study]. *Dtsch Med Wochenschr* 1984 Jun 22;109(25):987–90.

27. Fischer PA, et al. [Effects of intravenous administration of memantine in parkinsonian patients (author's transl)]. *Arzneimittelforschung* 1977 Jul;27(7): 1487–9.

28. Jain KK. Evaluation of memantine for neuroprotection in dementia. *Expert Opin Investig Drugs* 2000 Jun;9(6):1397–406.

29. Androsova LV, et al. [Akatinol memantin in Alzheimer's disease: clinico-immunological correlates]. *Zh Nevrol Psikhiatr Im S S Korsakova* 2000; 1 00(9):36–8.

30. Wenk GL, et al. No interaction of memantine with acetylcholinesterase inhibitors approved for clinical use. *Life Sci* 2000 Feb 11 ;66(12):1079–83.

31. Mobius HJ. Pharmacologic rationale for memantine in chronic cerebral hypoperfusion, especially vascular dementia. *Alzheimer's Dis Assoc Disord* 1999 Oct-Dec;13 Suppl 3:S172–8.

32. Parsons CG, et al. Memantine is a clinically well tolerated N-methyl-D-aspartate (NMDA) receptor antagonist—a review of preclinical data. *Neuropharmacology* 1999 Jun;38(6):735–67.

33. Ditzler K. Efficacy and tolerability of memantine in patients with dementia syndrome. A double-blind, placebo controlled trial. *Arzneimittelforschung* 1991 Aug;41 (8):773–80.

34. Huber Peter, "FDA Caution Can Be Deadly, Too." The *Wall Street Journal* 07/24/1 998 Page A14.

What's Wrong with the FDA

"That whenever any form of government becomes
destructive of these ends, it is the right of the people
to alter or abolish it."

THOMAS JEFFERSON,
Declaration of Independence, July 4, 1776

ONGRESSIONAL COMMITTEES and investigative journal-
ists have exposed massive incompetence, neglect
and fraud at the FDA. In the Courts, the agency
continues to lose critical cases as Federal judges rule that
FDA policies are blatantly unconstitutional.

For the past 21 years, the Life Extension Foundation®
has compiled evidence indicating that the FDA is the number one cause of death in the United States. The FDA causes
Americans to die by:

- Delaying the introduction of life-saving therapies
- Suppressing safe methods of preventing disease
- Causing the price of drugs to be so high that some
  Americans do without

- Denying Americans access to effective drugs approved in other countries
- Intimidating those who develop innovative methods to treat disease
- Approving lethal prescription drugs that kill
- Censoring medical information that would let consumers protect their health
- Censoring medical information that would better educate doctors
- Failing to protect the safety of our food
- Misleading the public about scientific methods to increase longevity

The greatest threat the FDA poses to our health is the fact that the agency functions as a roadblock to the development of breakthrough medical therapies. Innovation in medicine is stifled by FDA red tape, which is why Americans continue to die from diseases that long ago might have been cured if a free marketplace in drug development existed.

FDA Suffers Second Massive Legal Defeat in *Pearson v. Shalala II*

Court to FDA? The First Amendment Must Be Followed

I N 1999 THERE WAS AN UNPRECEDENTED LEGAL VICTORY against the FDA in a landmark Federal Appellate Court ruling. The title of the case was *Pearson v. Shalala*. For the purposes of this article, we will refer to the 1999 case as *"Pearson I."* When discussing the most recent triumph over FDA tyranny, this case will be called *"Pearson II."*

The historical significance of *Pearson I* cannot be overstated. By an 11–0 margin, an appellate court mandated that the FDA abide by the First Amendment (free speech) provisions of the United States Constitution. Prior to this ruling, the FDA behaved as if the First Amendment did not apply to them.

Still reeling from the devastating loss in *Pearson I*, the FDA on February 2, 2001, suffered yet another massive legal defeat in the *Pearson II* case. *Pearson I* and *II* are significant victories for freedom of informed choice in the healthcare marketplace. They make it clear that the First Amendment to the United States Constitution disarms FDA of any power to ban nutrient-disease claims (so-called "health claims") unless FDA has solid evidence that the claims actually mislead. The Courts have ordered FDA to stop censoring science on dietary supplement labels and to let that science reach consumers. The Courts ruled that the only constitutional right the FDA has on the issue of health claims is to insist on reasonably worded disclaimers such as, "These statements have not been evaluated by the Food and Drug Administration."

WHAT THE FDA WANTED TO CENSOR

In *Pearson II*, Durk Pearson, Sandy Shaw, the American Preventive Medical Association, Dr. Julian M. Whitaker and Pure Encapsulations, Inc. appealed an FDA ruling that would have prevented the public from learning that synthetic folic acid is more effective than food folate in reducing neural tube defects. The specific claim the FDA wanted to ban was:

> 800 mcg of folic acid is more effective in reducing the risk of neural tube defects than a lower amount in foods in common form.

In the *Pearson I* decision, the Federal Appellate Court ruled that the FDA had unconstitutionally suppressed this health claim. Over two years later, FDA still suppressed the claim in disobedient disregard of the *Pearson I* ruling. The FDA's decision to suppress this health claim not only violated the First Amendment rights of the *Pearson* plaintiffs, it also deprived the public of health information vital to every fertile American woman.

THE FDA IGNORES THE COURT'S RULING

The fact that synthetic folic acid in amounts ranging from 400 mcg to 800 mcg is more effective than food folate in reducing neural tube defects is well-established in the scientific literature. The Institutes of Medicine of the National Academy of Sciences has determined that synthetic folic acid is twice as bioavailable as food folate and, thus, is more effective in reducing neural tube defect risk. Despite the ruling in *Pearson I*, and despite the overwhelming scientific evidence in favor of the claim, the FDA held for a second time that the claim would not be allowed. In the process, it once again denied American women information they need to save them and their future children from the horrible affliction of neural tube defects. It also proved that this agency continues to be willing to harm the public health to keep in place its regime of censorship over health claims.

Pearson II is an outgrowth of *Pearson I*. A landmark First Amendment decision, *Pearson I* struck down as unconstitutional four FDA rules that suppressed the health claims that Durk Pearson, Sandy Shaw, the American Preventive Medical Association and Citizens for Health wanted to make. The four claims were:

1. Consumption of antioxidant vitamins may reduce the risk of certain kinds of cancers.
2. Consumption of fiber may reduce the risk of colorectal cancer.
3. Consumption of omega-3 fatty acids may reduce the risk of coronary heart disease.
4. 800 mcg of folic acid in a dietary supplement is more effective in reducing the risk of neural tube defects than a lower amount in foods in common form.

The Court also held FDA's interpretation of its health claims review standard unconstitutional. It ordered FDA to allow the four claims even if they failed to satisfy that review standard.

The Court ruled the FDA's health claim standard to be arbitrary and capricious because it was so subjective that no one could determine precisely what level of scientific evidence FDA expected in order to approve a claim. It ordered FDA to define a new standard comprehensibly—something that FDA has still not done. It told FDA that even in the presence of a defined standard the agency would be expected to allow health claims except in the narrowest of circumstances: when it proved with empirical evidence that a health claim was not only misleading to consumers but also that it could not be rendered non-misleading through the addition of a disclaimer. *Pearson I* made disclosure over suppression the order of the day. FDA was supposed to implement the decision immediately, fully and faithfully. FDA did not. In fact, FDA still has not done so.

FDA DRAGGED INTO COURT AGAIN

In *Pearson II*, Durk Pearson, Sandy Shaw and the other *Pearson* plaintiffs returned to federal court to force FDA to comply with *Pearson I* by allowing the plaintiffs' folic acid claim to enter the marketplace immediately. The Court granted the plaintiffs request for a preliminary injunction to the extent that it declared FDA's action unconstitutional. The Court held that "FDA acted unconstitutionally, and particularly in violation of the Court of Appeals decision in [*Pearson I*], in suppressing Plaintiffs' claim rather than proposing a clarifying disclaimer to accompany the Claim." FDA has sixty days to implement the decision but, rather than do that, it has asked the Court to reconsider its ruling, another delaying tactic.

Pearson II is a particularly bitter defeat for FDA because it comes at the hands of the very judge who ruled in favor of FDA in the case reversed by *Pearson I*: Judge Gladys Kessler of the US District Court for the District of Columbia. At oral argument before she ruled in *Pearson II*, Judge Kessler explained that she had been persuaded that her earlier decision had been incorrect. She said that she believed that the Court of Appeals' decision in *Pearson I* was the proper resolution of the matter. She then issued a very well-reasoned decision that constitutional law experts who have studied the case believe will be very hard, if not impossible, for FDA to appeal successfully.

In *Pearson II*, Judge Kessler rejected FDA's arguments one by one. She found FDA's failure to comply with the *Pearson I* order inexcusable, writing, "There is no question that the agency has acted with less than reasonable speed in this case; for example, it waited for more than 18 months before revoking rules declared unconstitutional by the Court of Appeals." She found it "clear that the FDA simply failed to comply with the constitutional guidelines outlined in Pearson." She stated that "The agency appears to have at best, misunderstood, and at worst, deliberately ignored, highly relevant portions of the Court of Appeals Opinion." She found that "FDA has continually refused to authorize the disclaimers suggested by the Court of Appeals—or any disclaimer, for that matter" and "has simply failed to adequately consider the teachings of Pearson: that the agency must shoulder a very heavy burden if it seeks to totally ban a particular health claim."

In granting the injunction against FDA's decision to prohibit the folic acid claim, Judge Kessler found, "FDA's decision . . . was arbitrary, capricious and an abuse of discretion." She thought it "very clear that Plaintiffs are harmed by the FDA's suppression of the Folic Acid Claim," explaining that the continued violation of their First Amendment rights constituted "irreparable harm."

JUDGE SAYS FDA'S POSITION "HARMED THE PUBLIC INTEREST"

Indeed, Judge Kessler found the FDA's suppression of the claim inexcusable not only because it deprived the Plaintiffs of their "rights to effectively communicate . . . health message[s] to consumers" but also because it harmed the public interest. FDA's existing, allowable folic acid claims convey the false and misleading impression that folate in unfortified foods is effective in reducing neural tube defects when, in fact, it has never been proven effective. The only source of folic acid proven effective is synthetic, i.e. the kind of folic acid found in supplements. The only amounts shown to reduce neural tube defects consistently and reliably are above 400 mcg, with 800 mcg regarded as an ideal dose by many leading scientists. The only large-scale placebo controlled clinical trial corroborating a 100% reduction in neural tube defects in women with no prior history of neural tube defect births involved use of dietary supplements containing 800 mcg a day of folic acid.[1] The FDA rejected this study, but Judge Kessler did not. She ruled FDA's rejection of the study an abuse of discretion, finding the need for the information substantial. Here is what the judge said:

> The public health risk from neural tube defects (NTD) is undeniably substantial. NTDs occur in approximately 1 of every 1,000 live births in the United States. Approximately 2,500 babies are

born every year with an NTD. Of the children born with NTDs, most do not survive into adulthood, and those who do experience severe handicaps. The lifetime health costs associated with spina bifida, the most common NTD, exceed $500,000, and the yearly costs in Social Security payments exceed $82 million.

Given that the scientific consensus, even as acknowledged by the FDA, confirms that taking folic acid substantially reduces a woman's risk of giving birth to an infant with a neural tube defect, the public interest is well served by permitting information about the folic acid/NTD connection to reach as wide a public audience as possible. Plaintiffs' Folic Acid Claim . . . communicates this vitally important message.

IS THE FDA NOW IN CONTEMPT OF COURT?

Pearson II and *Pearson I* have profound implications for FDA's regulation of health information. These decisions establish beyond any legal doubt that the FDA must comply with the First Amendment. Those decisions make it clear that FDA cannot suppress health information on the basis that the agency disagrees with the message communicated. Instead, FDA must be in the business of fostering the dissemination of health information to the public, not censoring it.

Although the *Pearson I* and *II* decisions concern dietary supplements, they rest on broad First Amendment doctrines that are the supreme law of the land and have greater authority than any FDA regulation. As a consequence, the *Pearson* decisions are likely to cause the toppling of FDA's censorship of food and drug claims over time. If applied to their full extent, the First Amendment principles of *Pearson* mean that FDA has no constitutional power to prevent the public from receiving any truthful and nonmisleading health information about any product that agency regulates.

Those principles mean that FDA must rely on corrective disclaimers, whenever possible, as an alternative to its current practice of censorship. The days of FDA censorship are destined to come to an end. For the moment, however, the agency still (even after *Pearson II*) continues to censor health claims for supplements, health claims for foods and off-label claims for drugs. That would appear to be contempt of court. In one case now pending before the United States Court of Appeals involving FDA suppression of a vitamin B6, vitamin B12, folic acid and vascular disease claim, plaintiffs represented by attorney Jonathan Emord have asked the US District Court to hold FDA in contempt for its noncompliance with the *Pearson* decision. It may well be that in due time FDA and its officers will be made to account personally for FDA's unlawful refusal to comply with the First Amendment.

Despite these incredible constitutional court victories, FDA censorship persists, as discussed when describing FDA's suppression of health claims about walnuts, cherries, green tea, etc.

Reference

1. "Prevention of the first occurrence of neural-tube defects by periconceptional vitamin supplementation," *New England Journal of Medicine*. 1992 Dec 24;327(26):1832–5.

MAY 2001

FDA Loses Case against Compounding Pharmacies on First Amendment Grounds

OST AMERICANS DON'T KNOW that they can legally obtain certain drugs that are not FDA-approved at compounding pharmacies. The cost of these "compounded" drugs is often lower than what it costs to buy finished drugs made by pharmaceutical companies. The reason most Americans don't know about drugs available at compounding pharmacies is that up till now, the FDA said it was "illegal" for compounding pharmacies to promote the drugs they offered.

A Federal appellate court has just ruled that the FDA cannot restrict advertising by pharmacists who sell compounded drugs. The decision pitted the free speech rights of pharmacists against a Federal law aimed at restricting advertising of compounds that require a doctor's prescription, but aren't subject to the FDA's approval process.

In citing previous cases, the US Court of Appeals for the Ninth Circuit Court (San Francisco) stated that "government prohibitions of truthful commercial messages are 'particularly dangerous' and deserve 'rigorous review.' "

In this case, the FDA contended that restrictions on ads for compounds were an attempt to balance the needs of individual patients with the protection of the broader public by "preventing widespread distribution of compounded drugs."

In an opinion (that upheld a lower court ruling), Judge Cynthia Holcomb Hall wrote that "the government neither explains nor supports" its contention that wider distribution of compounded drugs would endanger the public. "In fact, most of the evidence runs to the contrary," she wrote, noting that "compounding is not only legal under state law, but most states require their pharmacists to know how to compound."

Judge Hall went on to say that the government offered "no evidence demonstrating that its restrictions would succeed in striking the balance it claims is a substantial interest, or even protect the public health."

2000

Life Extension® Wins in the House and Senate

I N A STARTLING SETBACK to the FDA and the drug cartel, a bill that enables Americans to legally obtain lower cost prescription drugs from other countries passed the House of Representatives on June 29, 2000. This is great news for consumers who have been paying inflated prices for their medications because the FDA inappropriately blocked the importation of less expensive drugs from other countries.

The pharmaceutical industry's panicked response has been to run full-page newspaper ads stating that prescription drugs from Mexico and Canada are somehow "counterfeit" and cannot be trusted. This is a truly remarkable allegation when one considers that the lower priced drugs from Canada and Mexico are often manufactured by these very same pharmaceutical companies.

The drug industry is using scare tactics that have no basis in fact to block Americans from gaining access to lower-cost prescription medications, and the FDA wholeheartedly supports the drug companies. American citizens, on the other hand, are revolting against outrageously high drug prices.

On July 20, 2000, the Senate passed a similar bill—by a vote of 74 to 21—that allows pharmacists and wholesalers to import US-approved drugs available at lower prices overseas. The House bill, on the other hand, lets individuals buy drugs abroad, so a compromise measure is now being crafted.

CONVENTIONAL MEDICINE FAILS MOST AMERICANS

You might think that since US citizens pay the highest healthcare prices in the world, that the quality of medicine would be commensurate with the cost. According to the World Health Organization, this is not the case. A recently released study from the World Health Organization showed that the United States ranked 37th in overall healthcare quality, meaning that 36 countries are doing a better job than the US at keeping their citizens healthy. The fact that countries who are ahead of the United States pay significantly less in healthcare costs indicates that there is something fundamentally flawed about the present FDA-protected healthcare monopoly. According to a health economist at Princeton University, the United States is very good at employing heroic expensive procedures, but poor at low-cost preventative care that keeps citizens of other countries healthier. This is not surprising when one looks at the FDA's 80-year reign of terror against those involved in preventive medicine.

NEW ENGLAND JOURNAL OF MEDICINE ATTACKS PHARMACEUTICAL INDUSTRY

Anyone who reads the *New England Journal of Medicine* knows that this publication derives almost all of their advertising revenue from prescription drug advertising. That's what makes their blunt editorial against the pharmaceutical industry so credible.

This editorial, written by Dr. Marcia Angell, and published in the June 22, 2000 edition, accuses the pharmaceutical industry of hiding behind a cloak of "exaggerated or misleading" claims to justify high drug prices. Drug companies state that they need high prices to develop new cures and better treatments. But Angell argues that many of the new drugs that companies produce add little to therapeutic innovation except expense and confusion.

The *New England Journal of Medicine* editorial depicts the industry as one in which top companies rake in huge profits, spend enormous amounts on questionable marketing and advertising practices and are free to charge inflated prices as a result of government-sanctioned monopolies. "The pharmaceutical industry is extraordinarily privileged. It benefits enormously from publicly funded research, government-granted patents and large tax breaks, and it reaps lavish profits," says Dr. Angell.

Dr. Angell said that she is speaking out because the prices of drugs are rising so fast and the use of drugs is so great that it's becoming a real problem for consumers. She also worries that the ongoing Congressional debate on a Medicare prescription drug benefit has largely focused on who will pay and the breadth of coverage instead of the price of the drugs themselves.

It should not be surprising that the Pharmaceutical Research and Manufacturers of America, which represents drug companies, issued a prepared statement blasting Dr. Angell's point of view as "a complete distortion of the facts."

WALL STREET JOURNAL EXPOSES DRUG COMPANY PROPAGANDA

The July 6, 2000 issue of the *Wall Street Journal* also featured an article critical of the drug industry's claims that high drug prices are needed to fund research. According to this article, the pharmaceutical industry is not delivering the kind of breakthroughs that were once promised. The *Wall Street Journal* pointed out that the drug industry still spends far more on salesmen than it does on scientists and that overall, the industry's marketing and administration expenses are generally more than twice those of research and development. At Pfizer, for instance, marketing and administration make up 39% of expenses, compared with 17% for R&D.

WHY THESE ATROCITIES CONTINUE

Americans pay the highest prices in the world for substandard medical care. It's easy to point fingers at the drug companies, but it is the FDA who provides the pharmaceutical giants with the immoral monopoly that allows them to rape the American consumer's health and pocketbook. If the FDA were abolished, drug companies would have to get back to aggressive research and cut prices dramatically if they were to compete against the small biotech companies that are being held back by FDA red tape.

With the FDA out of the way, large and small companies would be free to offer novel therapies without having to spend hundreds of millions of dollars on FDA "approval." New drug efficacy would be determined by allowing private organizations to test drugs on volunteer terminally ill patients without first having to obtain FDA approval. In today's heavily regulated climate, on the other hand, terminally ill patients are denied access to promising therapies unless they meet the rigid criteria set by the FDA. This bureaucratic obstacle often dooms a drug to failure because the agency first demands the patients fail grueling rounds of toxic conventional therapy before being allowed to try the novel approach.

Some people still think the FDA protects us against dangerous drugs. Instead, when humanitarian FDA employees tried to alert the public about a dangerous drug, the FDA launched an internal affairs investigation and threatened these honorable people with imprisonment.

The FDA's primary focus is on protecting the profits of the large drug companies and not in safeguarding the consumer against dangerous drugs. It is encouraging that a growing number of judges, members of Congress and the media are recognizing the health fraud being perpetrated against the American public by the FDA.

UPDATE

Despite this drug importation bill passing in the House and Senate, the FDA nixed it on technical grounds. The result is hyper-inflated drug prices that are driving the United States into financial ruination.

In June 2011, Pfizer announced plans to cut $1 billion in research-and-development expenses for year 2012. This is on top of $2.9 billion in research-and-development cuts it previously announced. Pfizer has earned tens of billions of dollars of profits on drug sales. Yet their in-house research has failed to produce the major medical breakthroughs the pharmaceutical industry once promised from sales of their high-priced drugs.

MAY 2000

Americans are Getting Healthier—But the FDA Remains a Major Impediment

ACCORDING TO A NEW STUDY, life is not only becoming longer in the US, it appears to be getting better. People over age 84 in 1993 were shown to be healthier and more independent compared with those the same age in 1986. This new report was published in the *Journal of the American Medical Association* (January 26, 2000).

The study also showed that fewer men and women over age 84 used healthcare services and entered into nursing homes during the last year of their lives. According to a co-author of the report, Dr. Richard S. Cooper, "There have been substantial changes over the last generation in terms of health-related behaviors and we are beginning to see the impact of that among the elderly."

New studies are likely to continue to show significant prolongation of a healthier life span based on the aggressive measures Americans are taking to prevent the diseases of aging. One example of how Americans are taking better care of themselves can be seen in the explosive growth of vitamin supplements. Sales of dietary supplements in the United States in 1982 were only two billion dollars. By 1999, dietary supplement sales topped fifteen billion dollars. Based on the health and longevity effects that supplements confer on human populations, there should be increasing numbers of Americans who live independently, relatively free of the common degenerative diseases that have afflicted previous generations.

WHY THESE STATS ARE NOT GOOD ENOUGH

Improving the overall quality of life is a short-term objective of the Life Extension Foundation®. Our ultimate goal is the indefinite extension of the healthy human life span. There is strong scientific reason to believe that the eradication of killer diseases and control of human aging may be right around the corner. The problem is that an entire generation of Americans may perish waiting for the FDA to approve these breakthrough therapies.

There are biotech companies making revolutionary medical discoveries, but the FDA's regulatory quagmire prevents many of these potential life saving therapies from making it to market.We reprint on the next page an unsolicited letter that exemplifies the problem that small drug companies have in dealing with the FDA. This exceptionally well stated letter, detailing how the FDA stifles medical innovation, was sent to me by a biotech company president.

The solution to the FDA's bureaucratic obstruction of advancement in medicine is to radically restructure or abolish the agency. The dilemma is that the average person still thinks the FDA does what it is supposed to, i.e., "protect and promote the health of the American public." The unfortunate facts are that science is moving ahead too rapidly for any central bureaucracy to keep up with it all. The FDA roadblock against progress has to be dismantled or many more will die from a disease that could have been prevented or cured if free enterprise was allowed into the medical science arena.

A LOGICAL PROPOSAL TO END FDA TYRANNY

The letter below provides an inside look at how the FDA inhibits innovation and how simple it would be to restructure the agency in a way that would allow for a medical renaissance to occur in the United States.

From the Desk of
RODERIC M.K. DALE, PhD

February 25, 2000

William Faloon
Life Extension Foundation®
PO Box 229120
Hollywood, FL 33022

Dear Mr. Faloon:

I have read with great interest of your battles with the FDA. It would appear that the FDA believes that it is above the US constitution and that it can intimidate, threaten and enforce inherently flawed authoritarian regulations and even regulate what people can say. This last point was of course, documented in court in the lawsuit that was brought by Pearson and Shaw charging that the FDA was guilty of suppressing truthful and non-misleading information. As you know, the courts agreed with Pearson and Shaw and the appellate court voted 11 to zero not to hear an appeal by the FDA.

The frustration that our company has experienced stems from yet another aspect of the FDA's activities. Our company, Oligos Etc. Inc., is a contract manufacturer that has established itself as a premier source for the highest quality nucleic acids for research, diagnostics, nucleic acid arrays, cosmetics, nutritional supplements and therapeutics. Over the past several years we have been pursuing a research program using internally generated funds. These studies have led to the development of several truly innovative formulations based on our extensive experience with nucleic acid synthesis as well as novel chemistries and processes for the manufacture of nucleic acids that we have developed (patents pending). Therapeutic formulations of these compositions could be extremely valuable in inflammatory conditions such as psoriasis, asthma, arthritis, rosacea and eczema. Other compositions could be easily developed for issues ranging from hair loss, ED, IBD, cardiovascular function and cancer, to aging.

Originally we thought that we might pursue the development of clinical formulations of some of our compositions. However, we discovered that the therapeutic approval process that the FDA has created is extremely expensive ($200 to $500 Million) and incredibly time-consuming (8–12 years) for a single product. It is a process that allows only the large multinational drug companies to participate. Ultimately, a small company like ours would have to sell off its ideas to one of the pharma giants to get a product through the new drug application process (NDA). However, the large pharmas are resistant to new approaches. Even if they express interest in a new drug, they are as likely to bury it as they are to develop it, especially if it threatened to compete with one of their existing product lines. We spoke to numerous consultants including former FDA lawyers, business lawyers and officers of other biotech companies who recommended that from a business perspective we would be better off if we considered looking at cosmetic or dietary supplement formulations. This view was confirmed after seeing what happened to companies like Shaman Pharmaceuticals and Procyte. Both of these excellent biotech firms initially pursued clinical development of their products only to be frustrated, and eventually, after spending tens of millions of dollars, opted for nutritional supplement and cosmetic formulations, respectively.

As we began to look into the possibilities of other approaches we encountered the FDA regulations concerning cosmetics and nutritional supplements that essentially prevent the presentation of scientific research in support of product claims. We were astounded to find a US agency openly violating the first amendment right of free speech. The FDA has seemingly made itself the sole arbiter of what may be said in the US regarding food and drugs. As we began to read about healthcare in the USA it became apparent that the situation involved other players as well as the FDA.

The FDA working with the drug companies and the medical establishment has become a major impediment to both disease prevention and novel drug development and the principal cause of the horrendous medical costs both the country as a whole, as well as individuals, must bear. It is necessary to develop legislation to totally revamp the way we approach healthcare in the USA. The current medical system is basically not functioning well in disease prevention or drug development, and has flaws in the area of treatment while still costing a fortune. We do not need to spend more on healthcare. Those payments are basically subsidies for the major drug companies. The medical establishment has become largely an insensitive entity more interested in treating disease than in preventing or curing it. Please consider the following points.

As discussed above, the FDA has made the new drug approval process so expensive in both dollars and time as to preclude all but a small private club of very large and wealthy multinational pharmaceutical companies. The costs for drug development in Japan are reportedly about 10% of those in the US. This is not impossible to believe given that the cost for development of a new drug for the US veterinarian market is between $0.25 and $2.0 million. This is 1% or less of the cost to develop a drug for human use. It should be possible to develop new drugs for human use for similar costs.

At one time the documentation for a new drug application (NDA) would fill one or two 3-ring notebooks. Today, because of the FDA's approach that more data is always better, it is possible to fill an entire tractor-trailer with FDA mandated documentation.

Despite the exponential increase in all this expensive documentation, the number of adverse drug reactions (ADRs) to new drugs has remained essentially constant for the past 32 years according to an article in the April 14th, 1998 issue of the *Journal of American Medical Association*. The authors Bruce H. Pomeranz, MD, PhD and his colleagues at the University of Toronto, observed that ADRs to FDA approved drugs account for more than 100,000 deaths a year and are between the 4th and 6th leading cause of death in the United States. If one includes errors of administration the death toll may be 140,000 people per year (*JAMA* Vol.277, No. 4, January 22/29 1997, pp.301–306). According to the *New England Journal of Medicine* (Vol. 339, No. 25, December 17, 1998, pgs. 1851–1854), "Overall 51% of [FDA] approved drugs have serious side effects not detected prior to approval." Clearly, the FDA has succeeded in driving up the costs for new drug development while providing no more safety than existed when the costs were a fraction of today's costs.

Unfortunately, a triumvirate has developed among the FDA, multinational drug firms and the established medical community that benefits from perpetuation of the current situation. The large pharmaceutical companies begin giving "gifts" to future doctors while in medical school. (When is a Gift Not a Gift?, *JAMA*, January 19, 2000, Vol. 283, No. 3, pgs. 373–380). According to the *New York Times* (January 11, 1999, A1 "Fever Pitch: Getting Doctors to Prescribe is Big Business") over 6 billion dollars are spent every year to "educate" doctors about the new drugs developed by the large drug firms. The multinational drug companies also pay nearly $1 billion annually, in user fees to the FDA (The Durk Pearson and Sandy Shaw Life Extension® News, Vol. 3 No. 1, February 2000). As mentioned above, the costs for the studies required by the FDA can really only be covered by the big drug companies ensuring that the circle is complete.

The structure of the triumvirate is also such that what is addressed is the treatment of disease—not prevention or cure. The ideal drug product from the perspective of the large drug companies is one that is used daily for the rest of a person's life. For example, developing vaccines, unless needed yearly, is not interesting financially. There has also been a major effort by all the members of the triumvirate to restrict both information about alternative and preventive medical approaches as well as products such as nutritional supplements in the form of vitamins and herbal products. Long before it became open knowledge that the daily use of aspirin could lessen the chances of a heart attack it had been documented in clinical studies that this was the case. However, the FDA forbade manufacturers of aspirin from making those claims. It has been estimated that as many as 800,000 lives could have been saved over a 10 year period if this information had not been kept hidden by the FDA (Interview with Durk and Sandy, online at http://irc.lycaeum.org/~maverick/p&s.htm).

Another area that is truly absurd is the limitation the FDA places on the claims that can be made for supplements that pass through the intestinal tract. Although it has been shown that there is often better adsorption of nutritional supplements through the mucosal tissue in the mouth and nasal passages, according to the FDA, these routes of administration turn a dietary supplement into a drug. This goes under the heading of magic or perhaps madness. Likewise, although administration of many herbal remedies over the centuries has involved topical application of extracts, it is also forbidden by the FDA to make any claims if a supplement is applied to the skin. Again this regulation is clearly counterintuitive, but then the rules of logic do not seem to apply to FDA regulations.

The FDA, many doctors and the drug companies object to herbal and nutritional supplements arguing either that the herbalists and others are dishonest or that the reports are all anecdotal and have not been rigorously and scientifically shown to be beneficial. The FDA has therefore decreed that before any therapeutic claims can be made an herbal or supplement must be run through the FDA controlled $200—$500 million dollar drug approval processes. They also argue that people might forgo FDA approved medical treatment if they had ready access to alternative sources of medicinal treatment. Given the Adverse Drug Reaction data it could easily be argued that a person has a better chance at recovery and avoiding death if he or she avoids many of the FDA approved drugs. The former head of the FDA, Dr. Kessler asserted that, "The FDA should be the sole authority on health and nutrition." He also is reported to have said that if people were allowed to make health choices themselves there would be no need for the FDA. Exactly, and at that point people would have free access to information about ways to prevent many diseases, herbal and supplement therapies as well as novel approaches developed by innovative biotech firms, all for a fraction of the current healthcare costs. This brings up other points.

There are charlatans in every field, but that is hardly a reason for denying access to an entire area that has shown successes for several thousand years. Most medicines were initially derived from herbal remedies. After that most drugs were synthetic analogs of the compounds found in nature that appeared to be the active component. Unfortunately, pulling out one specific ingredient from a complex mixture can result in a toxic medicine. Many beneficial effects seen with herbal treatments may be the result of the interactions of several components. It is only relatively recently that the central approach to new drug development has lost all touch with botanical and other natural sources of medicines. The principal method of finding new drugs is to screen tens of thousands of chemically synthesized compounds in the hope of finding one that has the desired effect. As seen above, however, they frequently have other undesirable effects, such as death.

People are looking for non-allopathic medicinal solutions because modern medicine has become insensitive and distant to the people it ostensibly serves. Anyone knows this who has had the misfortune of either being in a hospital or having a loved one in a hospital. The alternatives frequently offered to people are a modern day version of the pit and pendulum. Given the large number of deaths due to adverse drug reactions, doctors, the FDA and the large drug companies' assertion that people need to get these treatments has a hollow self-serving ring. By contrast, there are very few deaths that can be attributed to nutritional supplements or herbal remedies.

If the costs for getting substances approved for medicinal use were not so exorbitant it would be economically feasible to take herbal treatments through the process. As it is, there are numerous excellent scientific studies showing both safety and efficacy that have been done outside the FDA arena. However, the FDA does not permit the inclusion of that data with the supplements.

There is a need for a new structure to handle drug development in the 21st century, one that is more open and far less costly. It might be well to restrict the FDA's activities to monitoring the food supply. A variety of ideas have been put forth. Perhaps the NIH and/or the CDC would establish standard tests for toxicity and a toxicity scale of 1 to 10 that would be included on every drug/supplement. The NIH could review the results of the studies, and assign a score to the particular drug. The company sponsoring the drug would then be able to conduct clinical efficacy studies. The cost of taking a new compound or herbal through the pipeline could be reduced to 1% or less of the current costs.

If it were possible to freely pursue alternative approaches to medicinal therapies that would include a healthy dose of preventive efforts, and include herbal and other supplements, and also to develop and market new drugs at lower costs, the entire crisis in healthcare costs could fade away. To restructure the current system will require formation of a coalition of the various groups involved in non-traditional approaches, as well as those opposed to the current drug regulatory process. These groups must pool their resources and efforts, join together and work with those members of congress interested in addressing the healthcare crisis to pass the appropriate legislation. If this happens we could see a new age of reduced healthcare costs coupled with improved health and longer more productive lives.

SUMMARY OF DR. DALE'S LETTER TO WILLIAM FALOON

The FDA, Drug Companies and the medical community derive mutually rewarding financial and control benefits from the current system. The triumvirate seems determined to fight any changes that would jeopardize their respective positions.

The current system has proven to be ineffective and counterproductive. It fails to address prevention and seeks treatments rather than cures for diseases, treatments that are often more dangerous than proven alternatives.

The costs associated with the system do not afford protection of the public from dangerous drugs but simply serve to ensure control of the system by the large pharmaceuticals, the medical community and the FDA.

The system has and continues to cost the lives of over 100,000 people per year in the USA.

The FDA, large drug companies and the medical community are the principal reason for the enormous healthcare costs that threaten the financial and physical health of the country.

While offering no solutions, the trio aggressively opposes freedom of individuals to pursue their own healthcare and the dissemination of truthful non-misleading scientific information about alternative and traditional medicines.

The current FDA drug approval process is so outrageously expensive that it prevents all but the inner circle of large drug companies from developing new drugs as well as making it too expensive to demonstrate the value of traditional medicines not covered by patents.

RECOMMENDATIONS

- Limit the FDA's authority to monitoring the safety of food and delete all drug regulatory activities from their charter.
- Ask the National Institutes of Health to establish a standardized series of toxicity studies with relative toxicity ratings from 1 to 10. All dietary supplements and drugs would be required to be evaluated and rated by independent labs and marked on labels.
- Let the FTC continue to judge whether the claims made for a product are properly substantiated.

BENEFITS

- Reduced healthcare costs—through reduced development costs of drugs and the use of alternative herbal and nutritional supplements.
- Improved health through prevention of disease. This also reduces costs and improves the quality and length of people's lives.
- A greater number of innovative drugs made available at far lower costs addressing not only the major diseases, but the aging process itself.

Sincerely,
RODERIC M. K. DALE, PhD

1999

The Plague of FDA Regulation

F EW PEOPLE REALIZE how long it takes before a scientific breakthrough turns into a life-saving therapy. The bureaucratic process is so burdensome that the total time from discovery to market approval has more than doubled since 1964, from 6.5 years to 14.8 years.[1]

One might think that this delay is at least providing Americans with safe medicines. The facts tell otherwise. This month's issue exposes a drug-approval system riddled with incompetence and corruption that results in the death of over 100,000 Americans every year from drugs the FDA says are safe. The current system provides a protected market for pharmaceutical giants who can afford to pay top dollar to get their drugs legalized in this country. As in any market that is artificially protected, innovation is stifled and the consumer pays a grossly inflated price for the final product.

The United States government officially endorses unfettered competition in the marketplace, yet when it comes to medicines, there is no free market. The revolving door between the FDA and multinational drug companies creates a system that excludes outsiders, and virtually ensures that Americans only have access to drugs guaranteed to make billions for large companies. The recent trend is for companies to develop "life-enhancing" drugs, such as Viagra®, at the expense of life-saving drugs that may return less profit. The FDA takes extraordinary steps to keep out foreign competition, even if the offshore drug is safer, cheaper, and more effective than its American counterpart. The net result is that Americans pay the highest prices in the world for pharmaceuticals. At the same time, we suffer the highest rate of drug-induced adverse reactions, in as much as deaths from prescription drugs are the fifth or sixth leading cause of death in the United States.[2] Inflated prices for bad products reflect a system that is corrupt and must be changed if Americans are to live healthier and longer.

Drug manufacturers criticize the FDA for the delay and high cost of getting new drugs through the system. One statistic drug companies point to is that from 1977 to 1996, they increased spending on new pharmaceutical compounds 15-fold, yet FDA approval of new drugs remained relatively flat.[3] Additional problems cited by the drug industry include turnover of FDA personnel, limitations of drug reviewers' technical knowledge and communication problems between the FDA and the drug companies.[4] However, large pharmaceutical companies are by no means innocent victims of FDA red tape.

All of this points to a bureaucratic quagmire that enables large drug companies to dominate the market, making it far too expensive for smaller companies to compete. But in a deregulated market, where economic success is predicated on a company developing effective products at a fair price, companies that make unsafe or ineffective products would be driven out of business, and Americans would soon gain access to more advanced medicines to prevent and treat the degenerative diseases of aging.

References

1. Advancing Medical Innovation: Health, Safety and the Role of Government in the 21st Century. *The Progress and Freedom Foundation*, 1996.

2. The *Journal of the American Medical Association (JAMA)*, April 15, 1998.

3. *Science* (1998:May).

4. University of California at San Diego study (1997).

1998

Life Extension® vs. the FDA a Hollow Victory: Why the Agency's Approval of Ribavirin is Inadequate

T HE US FOOD AND DRUG ADMINISTRATION has just approved ribavirin for the treatment of hepatitis C. Ribavirin is a drug that could save about 5,000 lives a year. However, 60,000 hepatitis C victims already have died while waiting for this drug to be approved, and many more Americans will perish because the FDA has only approved it for limited use. This is not the typical story about the FDA being too slow to approve lifesaving drugs. The circumstances surrounding this drug include several criminal investigations, felony indictments, stock market manipulation, squandered tax dollars, FDA agents traveling to

Europe, contamination of the nation's blood supply and lots of dead Americans.

The events began in the early 1980s, at a Southern California research laboratory, where scientists began taking ribavirin themselves when they contracted the flu. In most cases, their flu symptoms disappeared within 24 to 48 hours.

This was no ordinary research laboratory. It was partially funded by the Life Extension Foundation®, which meant that when the discovery was made, Foundation members learned about it quickly. In 1986, the Foundation recommended that members with serious viral diseases travel to Mexico to buy ribavirin, or order it from offshore mail order companies. The FDA did not like this (and similar recommendations we made) and, in 1991, the Foundation's officers were indicted on 28 criminal counts of conspiring to import unapproved drugs into the United States.

About the same time, the FDA also launched a criminal investigation against the New York Stock Exchange company, ICN Pharmaceuticals, that owned ribavirin, for the "crime" of promoting the use of ribavirin in adults. The FDA viewed this action as criminal because at that time it had approved ribavirin only to treat a viral infection that affects infants. Thus, ICN was charged with promoting an "unapproved" (for adults, that is) drug.

The FDA asked the Justice Department to impanel a federal grand jury to see if ICN officials should be charged with criminal misconduct. Shortly thereafter, the Securities and Exchange Commission also launched an investigation to determine if ICN had committed securities fraud by promoting ribavirin's anti-viral effects.

To avoid a felony indictment and avert financial disaster, ICN entered into a consent agreement to stop promoting ribavirin. The FDA scored a temporary victory by keeping ribavirin out of the hands of adults.

The FDA, however, was facing some serious problems of its own. Tens of thousands of Americans were contracting viral diseases from blood transfusions, and investigative reporters exposed the fact that the FDA had failed to protect the nation's blood supply. Of course, the media failed to appreciate that the FDA had kept itself busy by conducting record-breaking numbers of raids against vitamin companies, seizing personal-use shipments of drugs like ribavirin in the mails, and trying to throw people in jail for selling ribavirin to adults.

Not only was the FDA failing to inspect blood banks, but it also was dramatically reducing the number of food safety inspections. Meanwhile, tens of thousands of Americans continued to die from viral diseases that ribavirin was curing in other countries.

During this entire period, studies were appearing in major medical journals showing that ribavirin is effective against a wide range of viral diseases. Health ministries throughout the world were approving ribavirin as a broad-spectrum anti-viral drug. What made the FDA's stonewalling so serious was that there was no effective anti-viral drug approved in the US. Elderly people affected with influenza either got better on their own or died.

Influenza kills as many as 60,000 (mostly elderly) Americans in a bad year, and ribavirin stops many influenza viruses from replicating. While Third World countries were using ribavirin to treat their citizens infected with influenza, hepatitis and other viral diseases, American citizens were dying from these same diseases.

The irony is that many hepatitis C patients contracted their disease from contaminated blood that the FDA was supposed to have inspected. Rather than properly regulating blood banks, FDA bureaucrats choose instead to squander the agency's resources in an attempt to deny access to a drug (ribavirin) that could have saved the lives of hepatitis C patients.

Many of the hepatitis C patients who could have been saved by ribavirin are not dead yet, but their livers have suffered severe damage. While the FDA stonewalled the approval of ribavirin, these patients faced a significant risk of developing cirrhosis or liver cancer.

The Life Extension Foundation® never stopped informing its members about the anti-viral benefits of ribavirin. The criminal indictments against the Foundation's officers were dismissed in 1995 at the request of the Justice Department, but the FDA continued to harass Americans who imported ribavirin for their own personal use.

In 1997, FDA agents managed to convince European health ministries to raid companies that were shipping ribavirin to Americans for personal use . . . even though ribavirin was approved for sale to European citizens. The Foundation responded by launching a massive communications campaign to inform the public that the FDA had taken draconian steps to deny hepatitis C patients access to a drug that was shown to be a highly effective treatment against the disease when combined with interferon.

The most significant study shows that ribavirin combined with interferon is 10 times more effective in treating hepatitis C than interferon alone. The FDA's response was to instigate more raids against companies in Europe shipping ribavirin to Americans, thus condemning many hepatitis C patients to the permanent liver damage that often results in disability and death. (Do not use ribavirin to treat HIV infection. Ribavirin is not specific to HIV viruses.)

The economic cost to the Foundation for fighting for the approval of this one drug was enormous. Full page ads were taken out in newspapers, thousands of press releases were sent to the media, and hundreds of thousands of first-class letters were mailed urging Foundation supporters to protest the FDA's actions. The Foundation went so far as to produce and repeatedly air a half-hour TV infomercial attacking the FDA for failing to approve ribavirin and other lifesaving drugs that were already approved in other countries.

After 12 long years of battling the FDA, and after the needless, premature death of hundreds of thousands of Americans, ribavirin was finally approved. There still remains a significant problem, however: The FDA has restricted the use of ribavirin (sold in the US under the name Rebetol®) only to chronic hepatitis C patients who first fail to benefit from interferon alone.

Approximately four million Americans are chronically infected with the hepatitis C virus, according to the Centers for Disease Control. The CDC has estimated that 20 to 50 percent of chronically infected hepatitis C patients will develop liver cirrhosis, and 20 to 30 percent of those will go on to develop liver cancer or liver failure requiring a liver transplant. Hepatitis C infection contributes to the deaths of 8,000 to 10,000 Americans every year.

The FDA's approval of ribavirin is a hollow victory. After battling FDA bureaucrats for 12 years, most Americans are still being denied access to this lifesaving drug. Some people are actually applauding the FDA for approving ribavirin so fast.

In December 1997, massive political pressure forced the FDA to put ribavirin on the "fast-track," and seven months later, the FDA said that some hepatitis C patients can now use the drug legally. Somehow the hundreds of thousands of Americans who died waiting for FDA approval of the drug were forgotten.

A study published in the April 15, 1998, issue of the *Journal of the American Medical Association* (*JAMA*) showed that toxic side-effects from FDA-approved drugs are the fourth to sixth leading cause of death in the United States. This shocking fact exposes the FDA's failure to provide the public with safe medicines. The FDA-induced delay in approving ribavirin is irrefutable proof that the "drug lag" is causing Americans to die. Why is this irrefutable? Because, while the FDA itself now says that ribavirin is effective, history shows the FDA intentionally denied this lifesaving medicine to the public, to the point of spending millions of tax dollars trying to incarcerate those involved in promoting it.

FDA actions (and inactions) contribute to more premature deaths in the United States than any other cause. The agency routinely approves deadly, dangerous drugs that kill Americans, while failing to approve safe and effective lifesaving drugs for patients suffering from life-threatening diseases.

UPDATE

The FDA initially mandated that hepatitis C patients must first fail a grueling six month therapy period with recombinant interferon-alpha before they can try the ribavirin-plus-interferon combination therapy that was proven to work 10 times better than interferon by itself. The maker of ribavirin petitioned the FDA to allow more hepatitis patients to have access to ribavirin. The FDA capitulated and eventually allowed ribavirin to be used earlier in the disease process.

Epilogue

OUR GOVERNMENT HAS no idea what's destroying America's healthcare system. I doubt any elected official understands more than five percent of what you have just learned in this book.

One reason our political leaders wallow in blind ignorance is that healthcare is only one of hundreds of different issues they are responsible for.

The aggressive recommendations I have made for saving our nation from healthcare-induced insolvency are based solely on the factual data presented in these pages. The irrefutable fact is that radical overhaul of today's broken healthcare system is essential if we are to save this country from economic insolvency. Band-Aid approaches are no longer an option.

Those who read the financial news will recognize some of the harsh realities. Heavily indebted federal, state, and local governments can no longer afford healthcare entitlements, nor can individuals pay for them out of pocket. The reaction of politicians and bureaucrats is to point fingers as to who should pay more and who should receive less. It is not mathematically possible, however, for enough additional tax revenue to be collected, nor benefits reduced, to resolve this impending crisis.

Congress must enact legislation to allow free market forces to drive down sick-care costs, better enable disease prevention, and facilitate rapid development of improved medical therapies. This is the only realistic solution!

REBUTTING THE NAYSAYERS

Our healthcare system is like a country that has been invaded by a hostile foreign enemy. In order to successfully stave off an attack, there will inevitably be casualties, but that does not mean society should lie down and surrender.

To restore affordability, efficiency, and meaningful advancement to medical care, regulatory restructuring is mandatory—and there will be some casualties along the way. Analogous to the turmoil of the early 1980s when long distance phone calls were deregulated, there will be problems caused by regulatory restructuring (including deaths) that the news media will sensationalize.

But look at how fast telecommunications evolved—with technologies that would have been unimaginable prior to deregulation—and at a cost that has dropped so low that opening one's monthly phone bill can be done without trepidation.

Once the beneficial impact of healthcare deregulation occurs, the rewards will be enormous. For instance:

- Medical care will no longer be a major affordability issue for government, business, or ordinary Americans.
- Many common diseases today will be preventable, or at least postponed by decades.
- Better treatments and outright cures will be discovered for today's killer diseases.

REGULATORY REFORM IN A NUTSHELL

The regulatory restructuring required to reap these rewards is simple. Congress must pass laws that prohibit regulatory agencies (both federal and state) from taking enforcement action that impedes competition, drives up costs, stifles innovation, chills free speech, grants privileges to certain groups that are denied to others, mandates governmental approval or licensing, and creates wasteful and corrupt bureaucracy.

These seven fundamental changes to healthcare regulation must by enacted into law to drive down medical costs, while creating a scientific renaissance across the broad spectrum that we define today as "healthcare."

For example, the FDA should no longer be able to prohibit the sale of any drug, device, or other product that has undergone scientific testing but has not been formally approved as safe and effective based on FDA's current Byzantine standards, which as you have learned in this book, are an abysmal failure.

The FDA should also be prohibited from censoring claims about any food, dietary supplement, hormone, drug, device, or other product that is based on scientific study.

There is an important caveat. Liberating health sciences from today's archaic stranglehold does not mean that fraud or overt criminal activity should be tolerated. The difference is that those engaged in real criminal activity, such as hiding the dangers of lethal drugs, will be prosecuted, as opposed to threatening walnut and cherry growers who make health claims about their food on a website.

Any product or claim not recognized by FDA should have a disclaimer stating, "This product or the health claims relating to this product are not approved or recognized by the FDA. Use this product at your own risk."

To ignite this revolution, which will spare us the agonies of healthcare's financial collapse, we must first enlighten Congress to the absurdity of inane regulations that cause prescription drugs to be so outlandishly overpriced.

I ask each of you to log on to our legislative website at www.lef.org/lac to send your representative and two senators a letter that explains why drugs are so overpriced and how simple it is to enact legislation that will drive down drug prices by 80% or more. (A copy of this letter to Congress appears in Appendix B of this book.)

Prescription drug deregulation is just one piece of regulatory reform that Congress must implement. The advantage of making this the first counterattack against over-regulation is that savings will manifest rapidly. This will provide real world substantiation for Congress to implement the other free-market solutions described in this book to resolve today's healthcare cost crisis.

I hope that any rational individual who has read Pharmocracy will not let apathy stand in the way of political activism. Please log onto www.lef.org/lac to demand meaningful change that will save Medicare, Medicaid, and this nation's healthcare infrastructure from impending economic collapse.

Send This Book to Your Members of Congress

Governments collapse when ineptitude and corruption reach such egregious magnitudes that the citizenry has no choice but to revolt.

The book you have just read presents factual and irrefutable logic to reform today's broken healthcare system.

While *Pharmocracy* uncovers egregious FDA incompetence and abuse, Congress is the body of government that provides FDA with enabling laws that ultimately result in needless suffering and death . . . while the nation descends into financial ruination.

Implementing the free-market approaches advocated in this book could spare Medicare and Medicaid from insolvency, while significantly improving the health and productivity of the American public.

This book provides Congress with a rational basis to remove the suffocating compulsory aspect of healthcare regulation and allow free-market forces to compete against government-sanctioned medicine.

We believe if enough constituents send *Pharmocracy* to Congress, members of the House and Senate will be forced to read it and recognize the obvious free-market solutions to today's healthcare cost crisis.

For assistance in sending a copy of *Pharmocracy* to your Congressional representatives call 1-800-544-4440 or log on to www.LifeExtension.com/congress.

Send a Letter to Your Members of Congress

This letter may be copied from this book, or automatically sent to your members of Congress by logging on to www.lef.org/lac.

The Honorable _____
Washington, DC

Dear _____,

Enclosed are introductory chapters from a book called *Pharmocracy* that reveal how Congress can amend the law to resolve today's healthcare cost crisis and spare Medicare from insolvency.

As a first step, I urge you to introduce legislation that will enable GMP-certified manufacturing facilities to produce **generic prescription drugs** that do not have to undergo the excessive regulatory hurdles that force consumers to pay egregiously inflated prices for generic drugs.

The cost of prescription drugs is a significant contributing factor to today's healthcare cost crisis, a problem that threatens to bankrupt consumers and this nation's medical system. Passage of this common-sense legislation will quickly slash the cost of generic drugs so low that consumers could obtain them for less than what their co-pays currently are. This will save governmental and private health insurance programs, and ultimately consumers, enormous amounts of money.

Please don't be influenced by pessimistic alarmists who claim that less regulation automatically means more dangerous drugs. These kinds of scare tactics have been used for decades to force Americans to pay outlandish prices for their medications. And please don't be influenced by pharmaceutical lobbyists, who will do and say anything to protect their virtual monopoly over generic drug manufacturing.

The bottom line is that we as a nation can no longer afford to be bound by today's inefficient regulatory system that artificially inflates the cost of our prescription medications. The money is no longer there to support this bureaucratic morass, and you know that as well as anyone.

Kindly let me know how you plan to implement legislation that will help save this country from horrifically overpriced prescription drugs.

Sincerely,

Name: _____

Address: _____

Why You Should Join the Life Extension Foundation®

The Life Extension Foundation® is the world's largest anti-aging medicine organization. Since 1980, this non-profit group has uncovered validated methods to slow premature aging and treat degenerative disease.

A review of Life Extension's 31-year track record (www.lef.org/track) reveals it is decades ahead of mainstream medicine in identifying safer and more effective medical treatments.

Life Extension's expertise in combating difficult-to-treat diseases gives it unique insight into what's wrong with today's broken healthcare system and enables it to identify the common-sense solutions you have learned about by reading this book.

For over thirty years, the Life Extension Foundation® has exposed how over-regulation in the United States causes lifesaving medications to be delayed, or suppressed altogether. Life Extension has shown how this translates into extortionist costs to consumers, who are forced to overpay for what are often dangerous FDA-approved therapies.

It is vital that those who understand the urgent need to enact radical healthcare reform join the Life Extension Foundation®. There are over 170,000 individual Life Extension® members, along with millions more who read the monthly *Life Extension Magazine®*.

As a member, you can participate in the raging battle between vested interests that want to maintain their government-protected monopolies and those who recognize that meaningful free-market reform is the only way of keeping this nation from sinking into an economic abyss.

It costs $75 to become a Life Extension® member. Most join because they want to personally avail themselves of novel methods to protect their precious health. People also know that their membership dues and product purchases support scientific research aimed at finding cures for killer diseases and reversing the aging process.

You have just learned what changes are needed to spare the United States from financial insolvency. Your membership is vital because it is Life Extension® that is leading the charge against an entrenched medical establishment that will do virtually anything to prevent the free market from resolving today's healthcare cost crisis.

To join, call 1-866-580-8923, and mention code HCB— or visit www.lef.org .

Index

G

H